Springer

Milano
Berlin
Heidelberg
New York
Barcelona
Hong Kong
London
Paris
Singapore
Tokyo

Aldo Fortuna

Early Diagnosis in Neuro-oncology

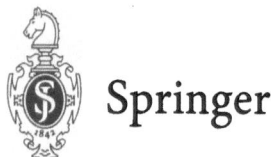 Springer

ALDO FORTUNA M.D.
Chairman of Neurosurgery
Director of the Neurosurgery Specialization School (1983-2001)
Department of Neurosciences
University of Rome "La Sapienza"

Note to the reader:
This book is being published also in Chinese

Springer-Verlag Italia
a member of BertelsmannSpringer Science+Business Media GmbH

© Springer-Verlag Italia, Milan 2002
Softcover reprint of the hardcover 1st edition 2002

Library of Congress Cataloging-in-Publication Data: Applied for

Cover design: Simona Colombo, Milan

ISBN- 13: 978-88-470-2212-6   e-ISBN- 13: 978-88-470-2210-2
DOI: 10.1007/ 978-88-470-2210-2

Preface

It is common knowledge that a clinical diagnosis is based on a combination of symptoms and signs, observed in their evolution; thus, every instrumental, laboratory, radiological, and electrophysiological diagnosis is based on positive findings of one or more report.

There is a stage of disease at which clinical features are scarce, but when an instrumental diagnosis, which is almost always the most useful, can be easily made on the condition that a diagnostic suspicion arises in an early stage of the disease.

This is particularly important for the neurosurgical clinical examination, in which early diagnostic suspicion means, in most cases, a timely diagnosis. The result is a drastic reduction in operative mortality and morbidity and thus a marked improvement in quality of life.

This work has a precise goal: to examine the "germ" of diagnostic suspicion, which is the true salt of medical art for every physician, general practitioner and specialist alike. In the following pages I also mention, when it is opportune, the characteristics of the late clinical picture: today, though, this must be considered as a medical failure.

November 2001
The Author

Contents

"Quia domini nostri sunt pauperes
quorum servos nos esse fatemur"

"As the poor are our lords
we recognize to be their servants"

Osp. S. Spirito in Saxia
Regula 3193 – Liber Regular C – CXXVII
Anno 1204

Biology and Pathology of Cerebral Tumors

In pathological conditions of the central nervous system (CNS), **neuroepithelial or intrinsic tumors**, which arise from cellular elements of the CNS and which are commonly called gliomas, must be distinguished from **benign extrinsic tumors**, which do not arise from neuroepithelial cells, grow in expansive form, and are noninfiltrating: these include meningiomas, neurinomas hemangioblastoma, and other rare tumors.

What are the possibilities and limitations of early diagnosis of epithelial tumors? A glioma can arise from a "mute" cerebral area, that is, an area without a sensorimotor function. This tumor manifests itself when it is large or voluminous. Unfortunately, this situation is commonly encountered by neurosurgeons. Generally, however, a glioma is discovered when, from a mute area, it infiltrates a cerebral area known as an important part of the brain, that is, an area with primary cortical functions. It is simple to understand that in most cases it is not possible to radically remove a glioma if it is extensive. Therefore, the great importance of early diagnosis in neurosurgery is evident. Today, destroying the "last" cell of a glioma is not an impossible goal. Advancing the diagnosis at an early stage would enhance the possibility of recovery.

We must underline that among benign tumors meningiomas are the most important and are seen most frequently. They are encapsulated connective tumors. Early diagnosis of meningiomas has two goals: to remove the lesion and preserve function.

In acoustic nerve neurinomas the importance of an early diagnosis is linked to the possibility of removing the neoplasm, preserving the function of the infiltrated nerve.

Therefore, the two most important aspects of an early diagnosis are that: (1) it is indispensable in extrinsic benign tumors both for recovery and to restore function – this also applies to some oncotypes of gliomas, such as cerebellar astrocytoma and ependymoma;

and (2) early diagnosis is at present the only possibility for initiating optimal surgical treatment of gliomas to prolong life, for as long as possible, preserving the CNS functions, and, in association with currently available antiblastic therapies, to achieve a definitive recovery in a very small number of cases.

Early Diagnosis
of Supratentorial Tumors

Prefrontal Tumors

Despite the use of modern neuroradiological tests, prefrontal tumors (those involving the part of frontal lobe located anteriorly to the ascending frontal gyrus) are rarely diagnosed at an early stage (Figs. 1-10). We often see the clinical-radiological picture of a voluminous lesion with manifest symptoms. Involvement of the frontal lobe is a serious situation and can greatly affect both the possibility of radical surgery and prognosis quod valetudinem. Hence early diagnosis is a necessity. Symptoms due to a frontal tumor frequently consist of the so-called frontal psychorganic syndrome. This is a psychopathic condition characterized by a triad of symptoms: dis-

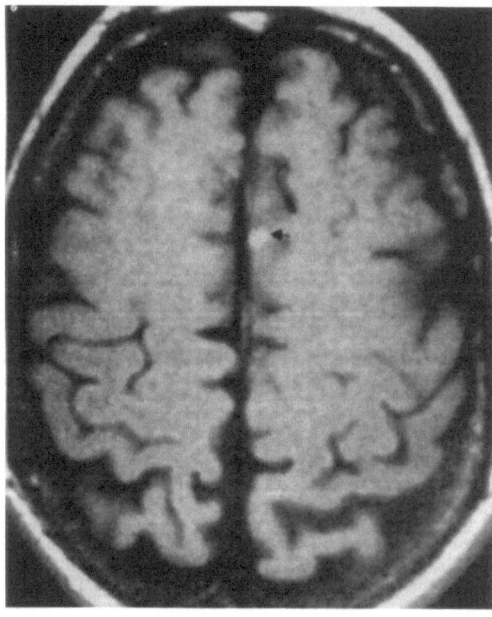

Fig. 1 Prefrontal parafalx left metastases: 3 mm. Axial T_1-weighted image following i.v. contrast enhancement (*arrow*)

orders of mood and character, disorders of activity and behavior, and intellectual disorders.

The mood disturbances have a slow and progressive course; thus, if they are not associated with other disorders, they are rarely helpful for making an early diagnosis. The presentation of these disorders varies, ranging from a "good mood", only considered pathological with difficulty or after careful observation of the relatives, to a dysthymic picture characterized above all by the use of obscene and facetious language. This disorder is called "frontal moria", consisting of excessive self-assurance, loquacity, affective indifference, joviality, and childish behavior. Another characteristic of this syndrome is disinhibition: the patients are not capable of critical judgments about their own social activities and behavior, which are restricted to playful, inappropriate language, often tending to sexual expressions, although the sexual potency of these patients is usually greatly reduced. The patients are unable to follow abstract logic and cannot cope with the problems arising in everyday life. Incongruous euphoria is often observed in the physician-patient relationship: patients are usually respectful and attentive to their physician but those patients with frontal tumors are uninhibited and often make scurrilous remarks about the physician and nurses. Euphoria often alternates with irritability. The patient resents any personal allusion and reacts violently to the slightest irony.

Motor activity disorders consist of hypokinesia, akinesia, and total or partial lack of responsiveness to environmental stimuli. There is no motor paralysis but the patient seems affected by a "mental paralysis of the limbs", with an inability to initiate action and work out the motor scheme. There is difficulty in initiating a marching step, which has a widened base and is characterized by short steps. From a psychodynamic point of view it seems that the patient becomes unable to change readily from one thought pattern to another until abulia and apathy develop and the patient isolates himself, answering only in monosyllables to show that he has understood.

Patients sometimes assume the typical posture of catatonia: the patient becomes immobilized for a considerable time in one posture or may maintain indefinitely the position in which his limbs were manipulated by the examiner. Generally, the patient accepts, without any reaction, the fact that he must undergo a serious oper-

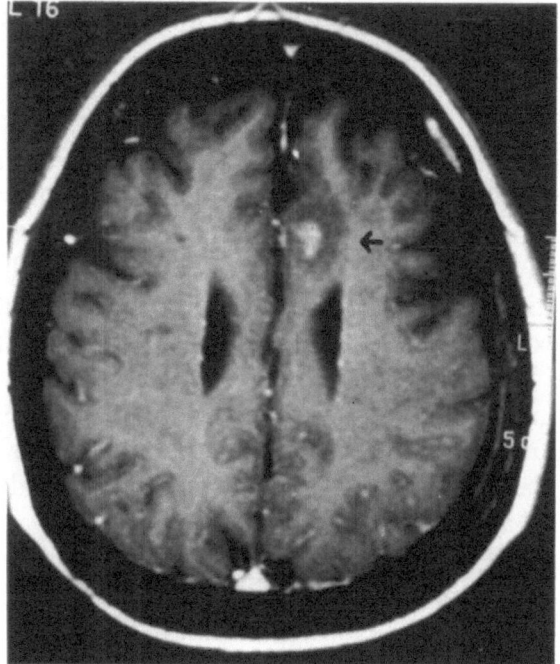

a

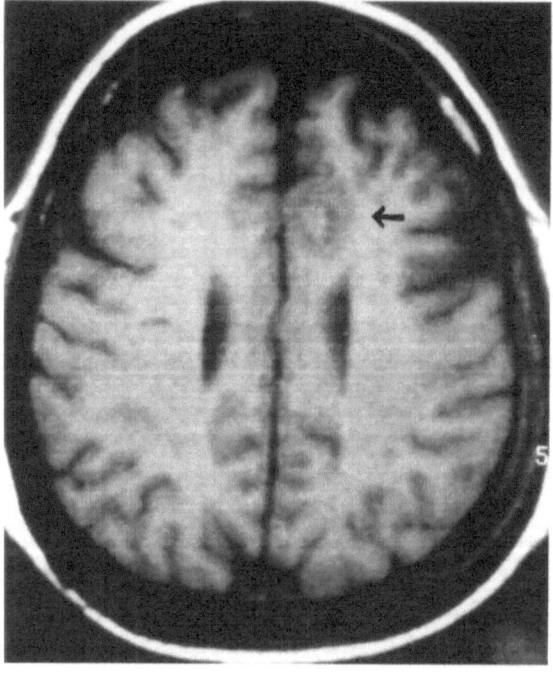

Fig. 2a,b Left prefrontal glioma: 10 mm. **a)** Axial T$_1$-weighted image following i.v. contrast enhancement (*arrow*). **b)** Axial T$_1$-weighted image, non-contrast study (*arrow*)

b

ation. The most common intellectual changes are attention and memory disturbances. These disorders are found in 60%-70% of cases; memory disturbances predominate (about 40%) and progress to affect the rational powers. Sometimes a tendency to pronation of the controlateral hand (pyramidal deficit) with hypotonia of the limb and flattening of the naso-labial groove can be observed.

Seizures characterized by conjugate head and limb deviation to the opposite side with or without generalization may also occur at the early stage. Epilepsy is a frequent symptom in prefrontal tumors. The patient often seeks medical treatment for this. However, the psychic disorders are insidious and underestimated at the early stage.

Epileptic seizures are the initial symptom in 30%-45% of cases and in the natural history of prefrontal tumors epilepsy appears in 50%-60% of cases. Seizures arising in the frontal lobe are divided into: loss of consciousness followed by a generalized convulsive state without localizing signs; loss of consciousness accompanied by turning of the head and eyes to the opposite side of the tumor; and adversive seizures with preservation of consciousness. These seizures are sometimes accompanied by an epigastric or psychic aura which can become generalized. The seizures with a psychic aura are characterized by so-called forced thinking. They are described by the patient in various ways: "forced to think about something," or "my thoughts suddenly become fixed." According to Penfield only adversive seizures with or without loss of consciousness are of localizing value, and they implicate the first and second frontal gyrus.

Changes in the superficial reflexes are seen early in the clinical evolution of tumors of the frontal lobe. Deep tendon reflexes are changed only when, in a late stage, the tumor extends to the ascending frontal gyrus. Abdominal cutaneous and plantar reflexes are altered by the tumor, and a grasp reflex may be seen. Abdominal cutaneous reflexes may be decreased or absent on the contralateral side. Loss or decrease of the ipsilateral plantar cutaneous reflex and a contralateral flexor response are of considerable diagnostic value (Botez).

The grasp reflex is characterized by slow flexion of the fingers after stimulation of the skin of the palm. Critchley (1927) stated:

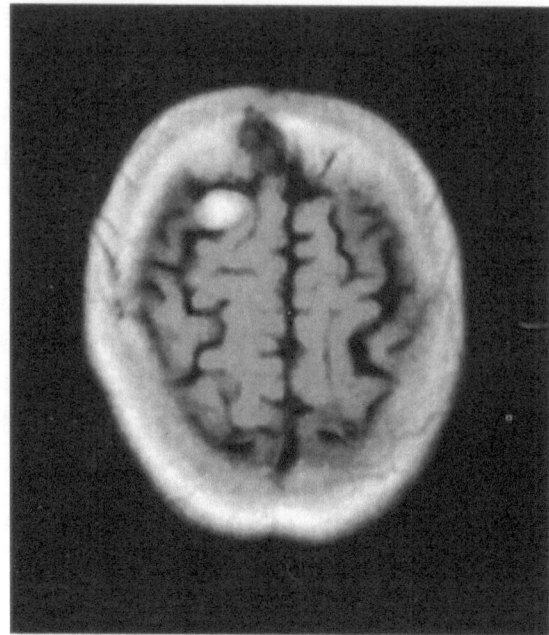

a

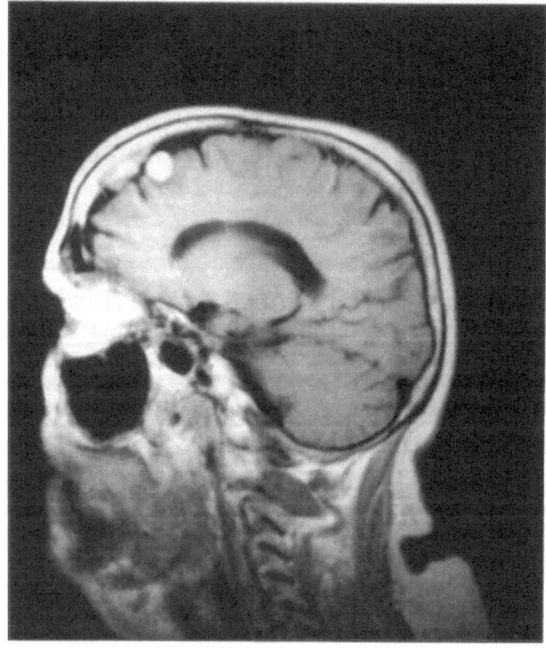

b

Fig. 3a,b Convexity frontal right meningioma: 15 mm. **a)** Axial T_1-weighted image following i.v. contrast enhancement. **b)** Sagittal T_1-weighted image following i.v. contrast enhancement

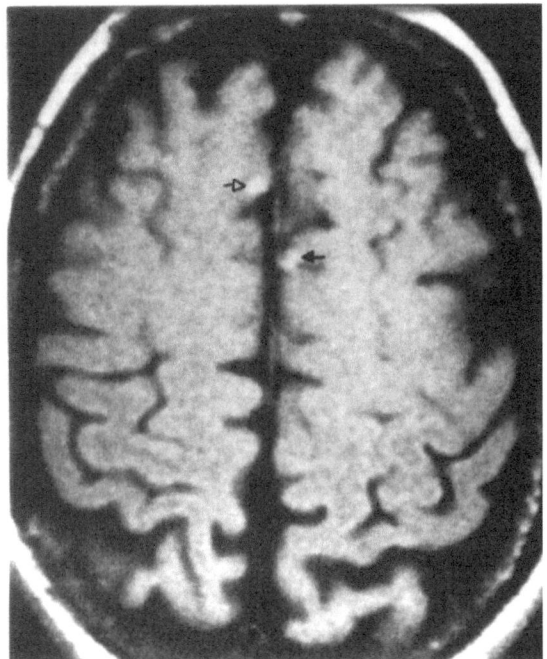

a

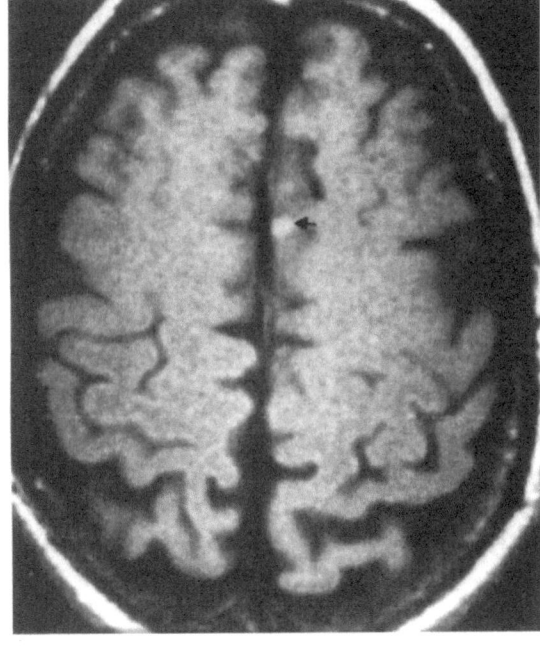

b

Fig. 4a,b Multiple frontal left metastasis: 3-4 mm. **a)** Axial T_1-weighted image following i.v. contrast enhancement (*arrows*). **b)** Frontal parafalx left metastases: 3 mm. Axial T_1-weighted image following i.v. contrast enhancement (*arrow*)

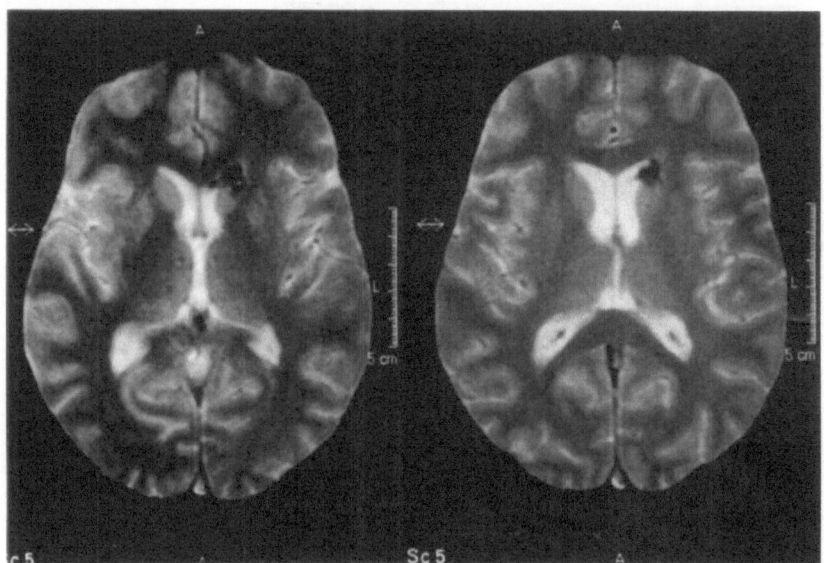

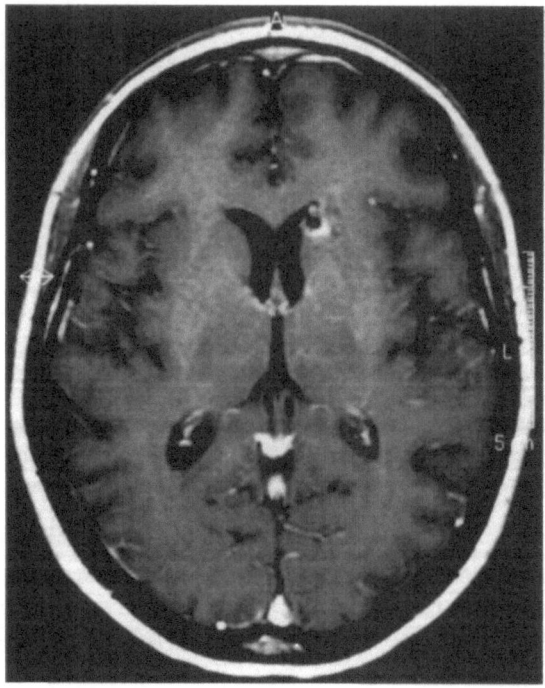

Fig. 5a,b Cavernous angioma left frontal horn: 8 mm. **a)** Axial GE image showing hypointense lesion. **b)** Axial T_1-weighted image following i.v. contrast enhancement

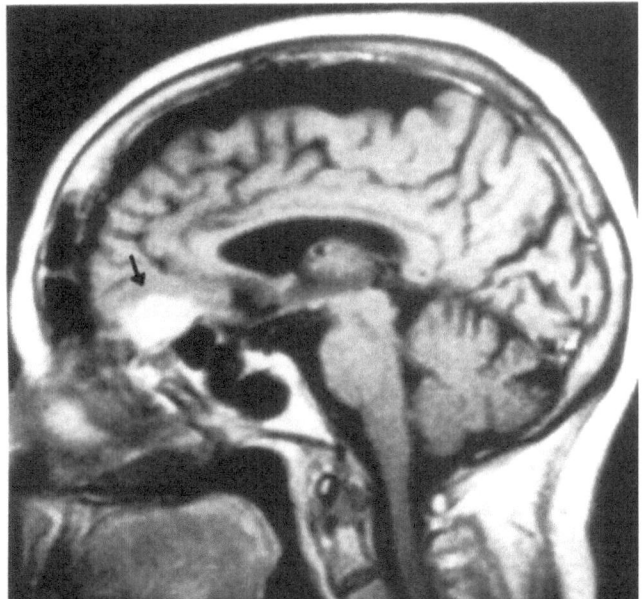

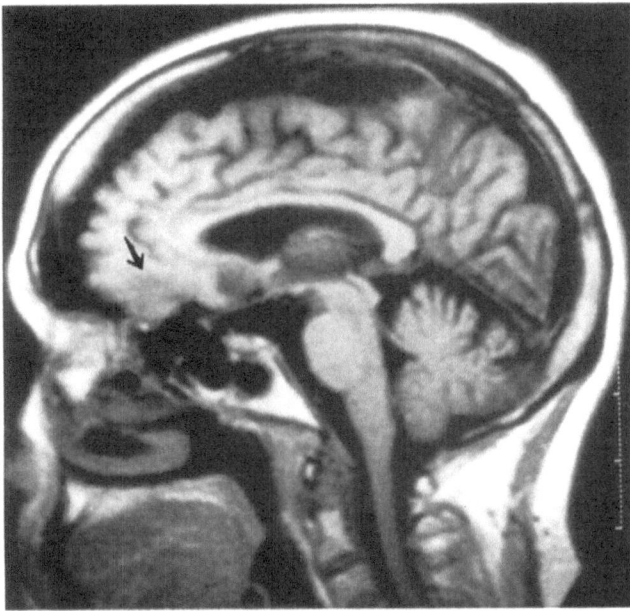

Fig. 6a,b Olfactory groove meningioma: 20 mm. **a)** Sagittal T₁-weighted image following i.v. contrast enhancement. **b)** Sagittal T₁-weighted image, noncontrast study

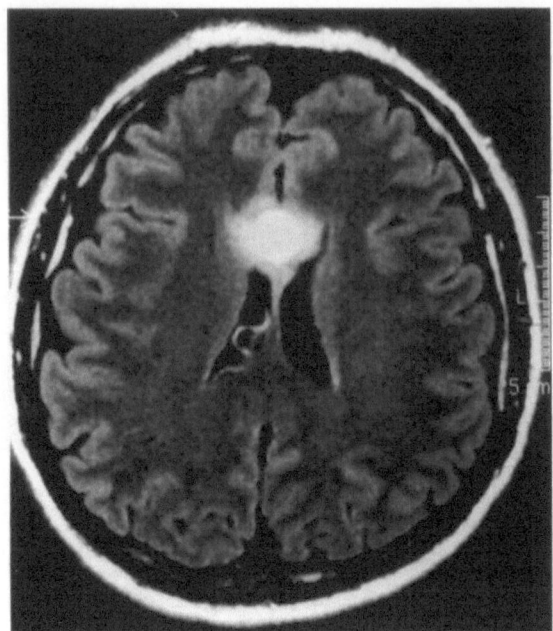

a

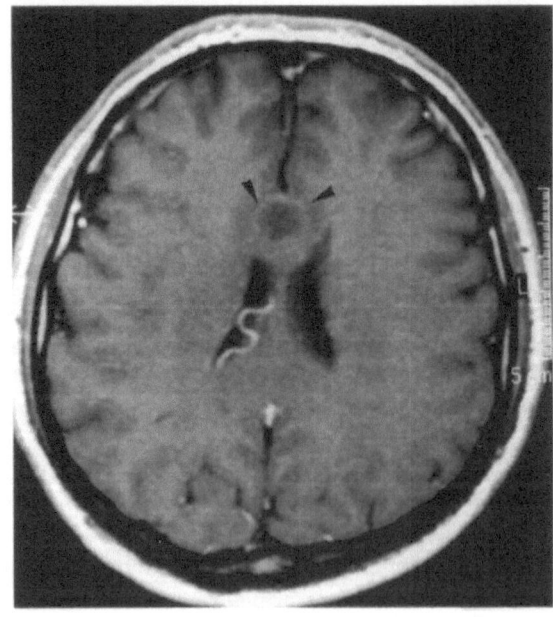

Fig. 7a,b Corpus callosum lymphoma: 17 mm. **a)** Axial FLAIR image showing hyperintensity of the lesion. **b)** Axial T$_1$-weighted image following i.v. contrast enhancement (*arrows*)

b

"their presence (grasp reflex) in a patient with a cerebral tumor is unequivocal evidence of the situation of the tumor in the frontal lobe on the side opposite to the hand showing the grasp reflex". Sager (1950) concluded that, if the tonic component of the grasp reflex is strictly unilateral, its appearance is due to a lesion in the heterolateral Brodmann's area 6. The tonic palm reflex (adduction and slight flexion of the thumb after stimulation along a palm fold with a sharp object) is of value in localising a lesion only if it is unilateral. Both the Mayer-Reisch phenomenon and the Potzl phenomenon, i.e., persistent contration of the quadriceps femoris during passive flexion of the hip on the pelvis, plus a tonic extension of the digits are further signs of a frontal tumor.

Two further reflexes may also reveal the presence of a tumor in the frontal lobe: a pollicomental reflex (contraction of the ipsilateral mentalis muscle elicited by stroking the volar surface of the terminal phalanx of the thumb) and the finger-tip thumb reflex (extension of the thumb evoked by pressure on the second, third, and fourth digits).

Precentral Tumors

Tumors involving the precentral area (ascending frontal gyrus), unlike prefrontal tumors, are diagnosed in an early stage because of their effects on the motor cortex. Tumors localized in precentral area, though small, produce contralateral Jacksonian fits. Localization of the critical area depends on the cortical irritation point in the gyrus and can involve the contralateral side of the face or body.

A typical Jacksonian seizure may be followed by a transitory paralysis of the involved limb (postconvulsive paralysis). This paralysis lasts from a few minutes to 24 h and is attributed to functional exhaustion of the involved nerve cells, showing electrophysiologic signs of an absolutely refractory period. The histologic type of cerebral tumors is not correlated with the incidence of Jacksonian seizures, but epileptic seizures often occur in patients with cerebral metastases. Jacksonian seizures are generally followed by motor deficit in a late stage of the disease. Precentral tumors involving the foot of the third frontal gyrus, in the dominant hemisphere, cause speech disorders. These signs are important for early diagnosis. Speech defects are characterized by motor aphasia which is preceded or followed by spasmodic arrest of speech and vocalization fits.

Parietal Lobe Tumors

A focal epileptic crisis can be the first symptom of a parietal tumor (Figs. 8, 9). This symptom is reported in 50% of cases. Typically the crisis is characterized by paroxysmal paresthesia as a sensation of pins and needles or numbness in the contralateralside of the body, followed – or not – by Jacksonian-type fits. The crisis only rarely develops into a generalized convulsion (10% of cases). From a histological point of view epileptic crises due to parietal tumors have important diagnostic value because they occur more frequently in meningiomas.

Generally, nonictal sensory disturbances follow Jacksonian crises. They occur preferentially in more anteriorly located parietal tumors, and less so in parietotemporal or parieto-occipital tumors. Initially, the patient has a sensation of tingling or electric current of the upper extremity, one side of the face, or (more rarely) the whole contralateral half of the body. These disorders are accompanied by deep sensation disturbances, with a similar distribution, such as astereognosis and tactile discrimination. These disorders can cause difficulty or incoordination of movement. However there are no motor disturbances which can be objectively confirmed. A valuable early sign of involvement of the ascending parietal gyrus is sensory loss on the side of the body contralateral to the tumor. Patients who do not have hypoesthesia neglect the contralateral stimulus when both sides of the body are stimulated simultaneously.

From a neuropsychological point of view, parietal tumors cause agnosia, apraxia, and aphasia. Agnosia is a deficit in which an object or body parts cannot be identified in space. There are various types of agnosia: anosognosia (agnosia of one's own disease); and in about 50% of parietal tumors, especially in the nondominant hemisphere, somatognosia, the inability to recognize the half of one's own body contralateral to the lesion, in which case the tumor would be extensive. In lesions of the dominant hemisphere, especially in the region

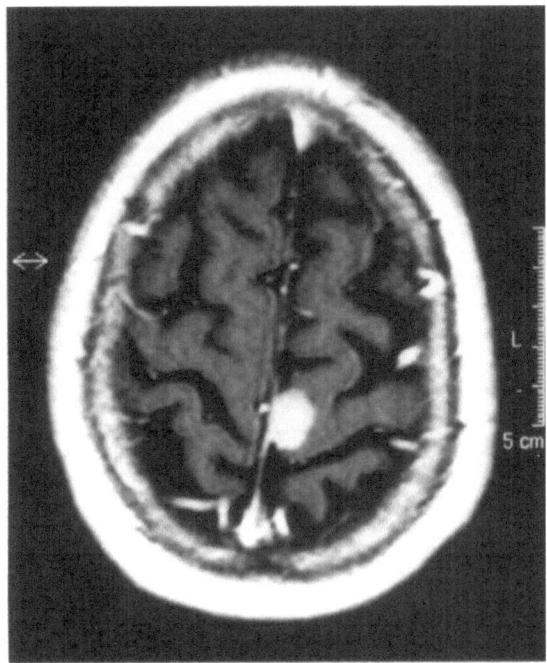

a

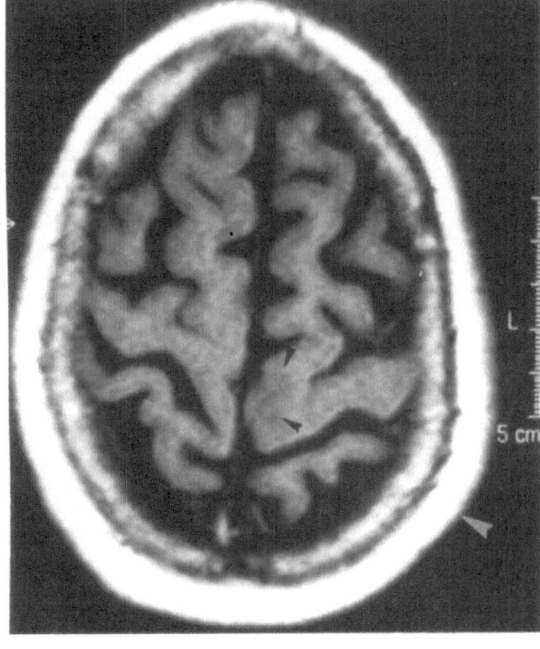

b

Fig. 8a,b Left falx meningioma: 12 mm. **a)** Axial T_1-weighted image following i.v. contrast enhancement. **b)** Axial T_1-weighted image, noncontrast study (*arrows*)

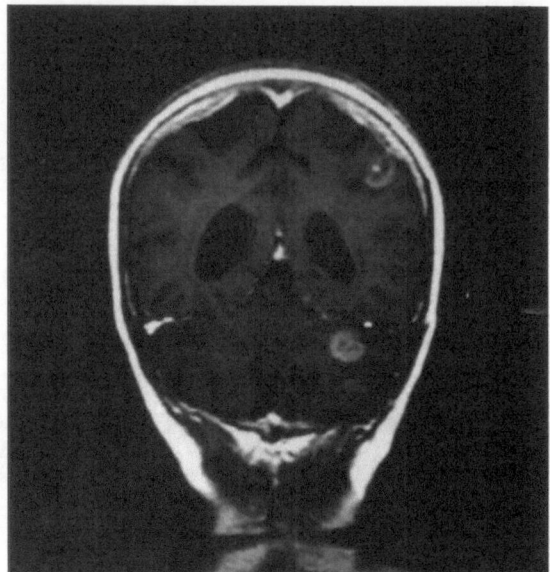

a

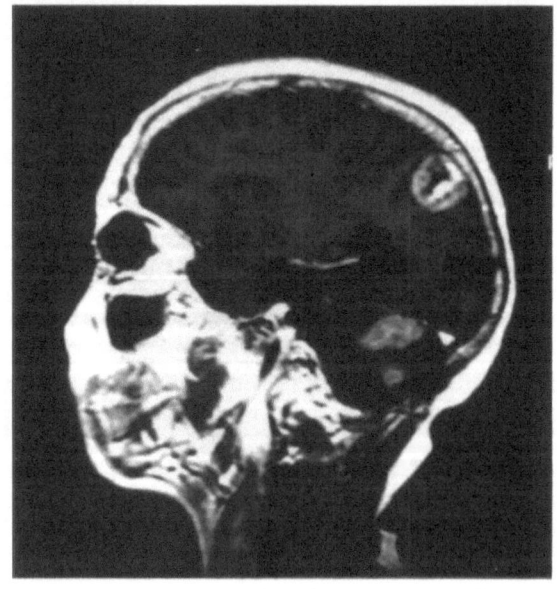

Fig. 9a,b Multiple metastasis: 10 mm. (parietal and cerebellar). **a)** Coronal T$_1$-weighted image following i.v. contrast enhancement. **b)** Same case. Sagittal T$_1$-weighted image following i.v. contrast enhancement

b

of the angular gyrus, finger agnosia may occur with right-left orientation disturbances.

These body scheme disorders in combination with agraphia and acalculia are known as Gerstmann's syndrome. Apraxia involves the inability to identify a motor act, without motor deficits. This is due to a loss of the logical processes that are necessary to execute the correct sequence of simple movements which constitute the complex act. Apraxia alone in parietal lobe tumors is rare. Frequently, it occurs as an inability to draw or as a writing disorder. This is present in tumors of the dominant hemisphere and is due both to pure apraxia (i.e., agraphia) and to neglect of the contralateral visual field.

Temporal Lobe Tumors

The nervous structures of the temporal lobe are very epileptogenic; therefore, signs of a small tumor may be revealed early as epileptic crises (Fig. 10).

The incidence of epilepsy in temporal lobe tumors is high (about 50% of cases), being the first symptom in 34% of cases. Psychomotor crises are characterized by a slight impairment of consciousness (dreamy state), accompanied by behavioral and psychic disorders. Mental disorders may present as depersonalization or déjà-vu, sometimes associated with auditory or visual hallucinations and stereotypic motor behavior (chewing movements, repetitive gestures) or complex and pseudo-purposeful acts (i.e., to execute all sequential acts for an action, also very complex).

In addition, abrupt changes in mood can occur, such as sudden anger, depression, or elation (so-called gelastic epilepsy). These crises can appear as an independent symptom or constitute the aura of a generalized epileptic attack. Such crises are more frequent in slow-growing tumors and their incidence is twice as high in oligodendrogliomas and astrocytomas as in glioblastoma multiforme.

Olfactory and gustatory hallucinations are reported as the first symptom in 15% of patients. These symptoms are helpful in early diagnosis. Other phenomena related to these senses are prolonged preservation and distortion of smell or taste sensations. These symptoms can constitute the aura to epileptic seizures: they are

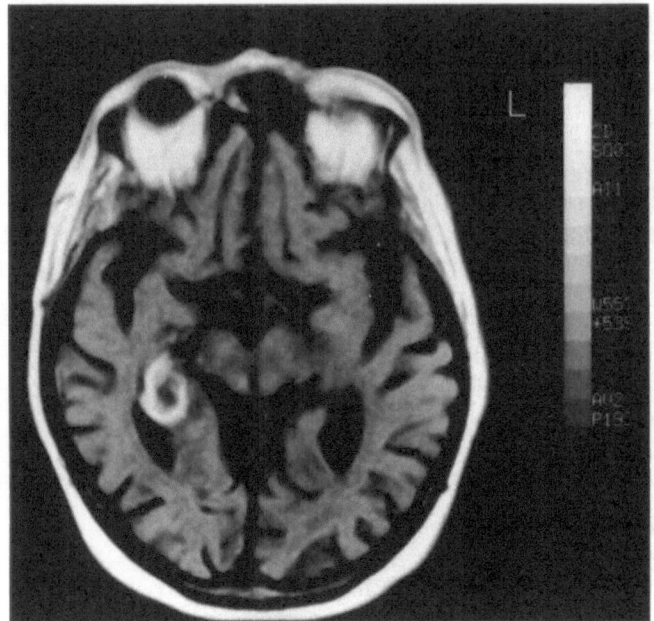

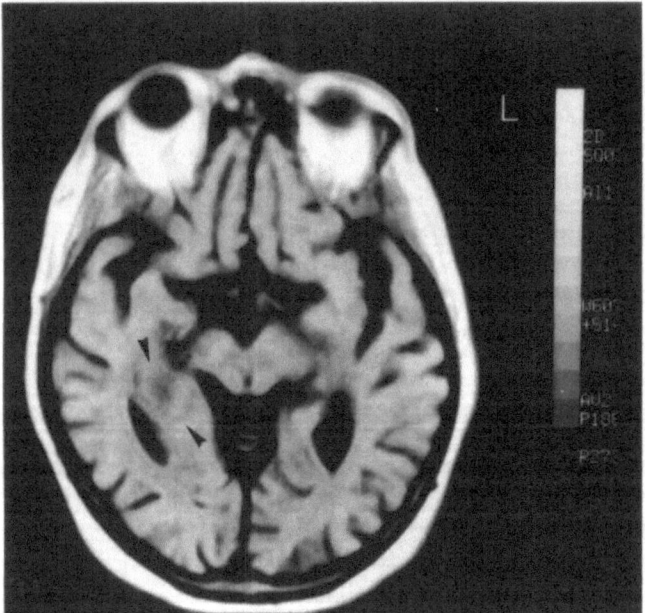

Fig. 10a,b Right trigone glioma: 15 mm. **a)** Axial T_1-weighted image following i.v. contrast enhancement. **b)** Axial T_1-weighted image, noncontrast study (*arrows*)

often persistent and can appear as an independent symptom, but then they are frequently followed by epileptic attacks.

The auditory sense is represented in the temporal cortex, but impairment of hearing or tinnitus is rare. Visual field defects occur frequently; however, this disorder occurs in a late stage of disease due to the involvement of the optic radiations rather than of the cellular bodies. Homonymous quadrantanopia of the upper quadrants is an early symptom of temporal tumors with medial development. Language disorder is a typical symptom. Aphasia presents initially as a nominal aphasia. The patient speaks fluently, but has difficulty in finding the name of the objects. When offered the proper term, the patient can continue speaking intelligibly. Aphasia can be the first symptom of a temporal tumor of the dominant hemisphere, but it often occurs when the tumor is extensive. Receptive aphasia represents ulterior evolution of the language disorder. This is due to involvement of the angular and supramarginal gyri and is characterized by an inability to comprehend words. This is not helpful for an early diagnosis because it occurs in extensive involvement of the temporal lobe.

Early clinical diagnosis of temporal tumors is possible when the tumor causes irritative symptoms during the initial growth phase. The disorders due to deficit of lobe function (i.e., aphasia) occur when the tumor extensively involves the lobe.

Occipital Lobe Tumors

The infrequency of tumors of the occipital lobe is in relation to the small volume of the occipital lobe (3%-4% of the total group of supratentorial tumors) (Fig. 11).

Focal seizures can occur early. Visual hallucinations are present in 15%-25% of cases. A focal seizure is generally an elementary visual hallucination (colored or luminous globes, lines, points, or disks) in a direction from the periphery to the center of the visual field.

These events can be preceded by conjugate deviation of the eyes to the opposite side and nystagmus. If the tumor has extended to the temporal lobe, the hallucinations become complex, including figures and scenes. Visual hallucinations, which can constitute a focal

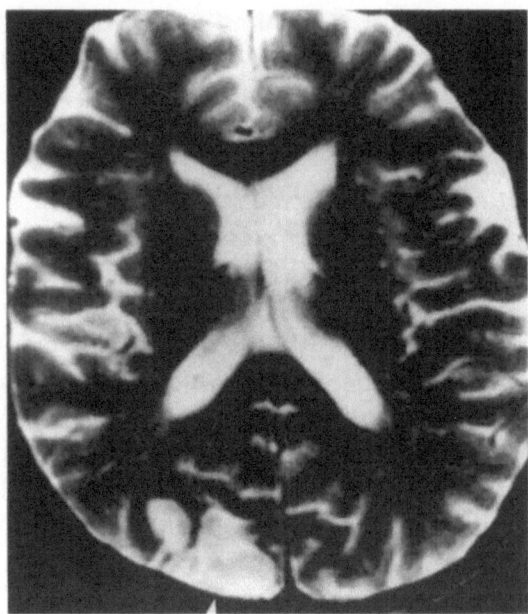

a

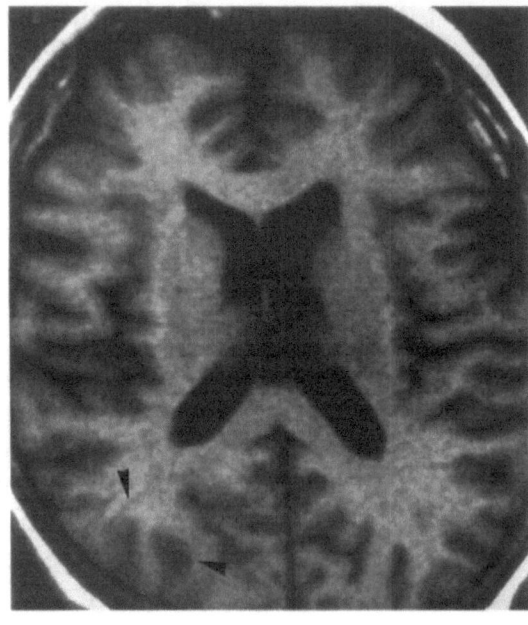

Fig. 11a,b Occipital right strocytoma: 20 mm. **a)** Axial T_2-weighted image showing hyperintense lesion. **b)** Same case. Axial T_1-weighted image showing hypointense lesion (*arrows*)

b

seizure or an aura of a generalized epileptic attack, can occur as an isolated symptom in a late stage of disease.

Visual field defects such as a contralateral homonymous hemianopia develop after epilepsy, but they can also appear in small tumors.

In relation to the side of the lesion, differential diagnosis of homonymous hemianopia is between occipital tumors and those of the optic tract and optic radiations.

The visual field defect associated with occipital lobe tumors is frequently extensive. Two characteristics are important for differential diagnosis: (1) the visual field defect is congruous and equal in two hemifields (contralateral nasal and homolateral temporal). The incongruity is related to the homolateral temporal crescent only (sparing of the temporal crescent is suggestive of a lesion located anteriorly to the cortical visual area) (2). Lateral homonymous hemianopia is associated with macular sparing. The physiopathology of macular sparing is still under study but seems to be due to a cortical bilateral representation of vision in the maculae.

Another sign of occipital lobe tumors is a color vision disturbance. A color perception disorder can precede hemianopia. This disorder is characterized by blurring of vision and a delay in the recognition of colors (so-called cerebral asthenopia for colors). In a late stage a loss in the capacity to visualize colors may be found and the patient sees entities in different shades of gray. Another symptom is visual agnosia, a deficit in which an object cannot be identified by means of sight even though the patient's tactile sense and visual acuity or visual field is not affected. There are several varieties of visual agnosia: defective recognition of objects (visual objects agnosia); impaired recognition of colors (color agnosia) or of spatial relationships (visuo-spatial agnosia); or defective identification of faces (prosopagnosia). Individual elements of a picture may be recognized, but not the meaning of the total picture (simultagnosia). Agnosia is often associated with a visual memory deficit. The association of psycho-visual disorders and loss of dream activity is termed Charcot-Wilbrand syndrome. This syndrome can be observed in occipital lobe tumors and is due to an interruption of pathways between the visual cortex and visual memory in Brodman's areas 18 and 19.

Sellar and Parasellar Tumors

In relation to the involvement of the optic chiasm, it is important to mention the possible locations of sellar and parasellar tumors (Fig. 12). In most cases they are situated above the sellar diaphragm (normal fixed chiasms), at the sellar tubercle level (prefixed chiasm), or above the sellar dorsum (postfixed chiasm).

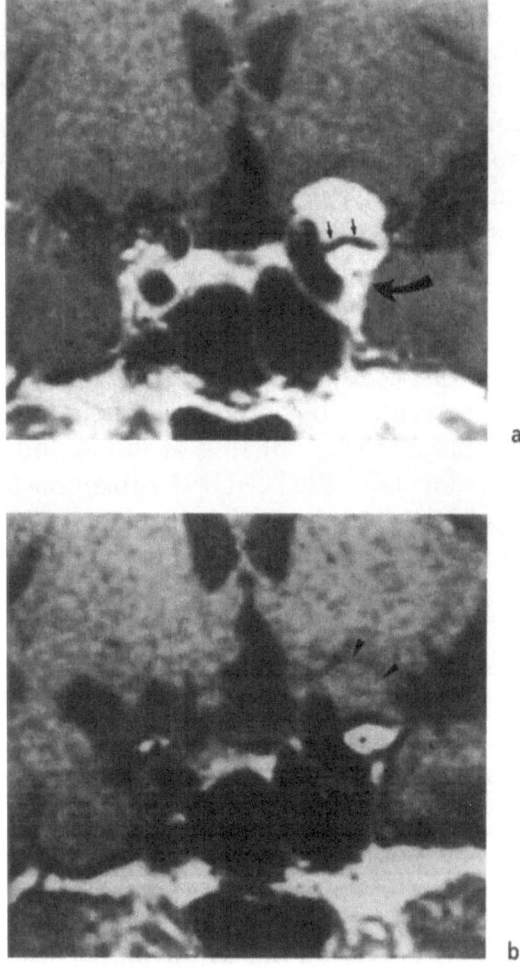

Fig. 12a-f Parasellar left meningioma: 13 mm. **a)** Coronal T_1-weighted image following i.v. contrast enhancement involving cavernous sinus and branch of the carotid artery (*arrows*). **b)** Same image, noncontrast study (*arrows*) ⟶

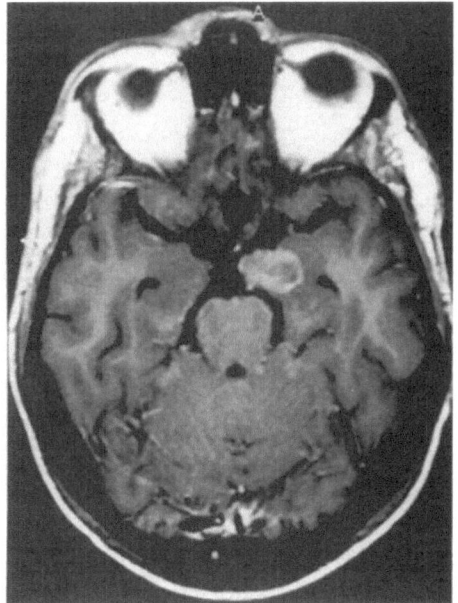

c

d

Fig. 12c,d Parasellar left metastases: 16 mm. **c)** Axial T$_1$-weighted image following i.v. contrast enhancement. **d)** Axial T$_1$-weighted image, noncontrast study ⟶

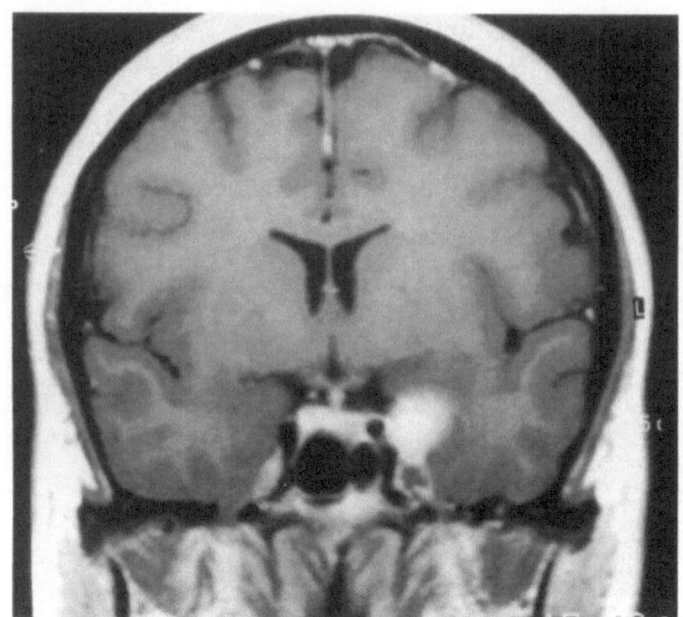

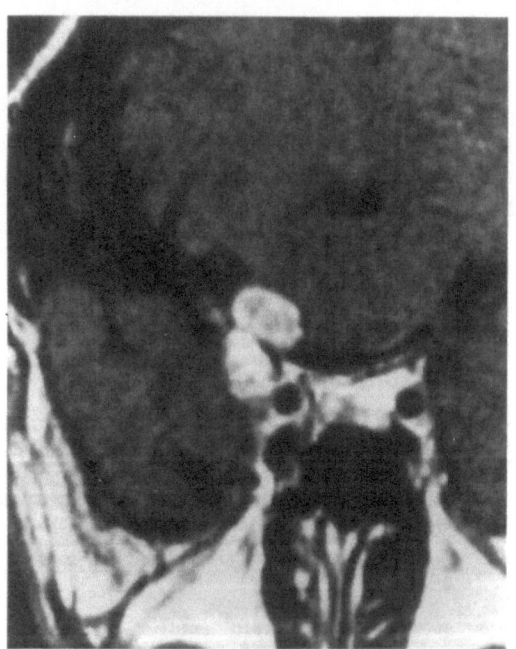

Fig. 12e,f Left trigeminal nerve neurinoma: 15 mm. **e)** Axial T$_1$-weighted image following i.v. contrast enhancement. **f)** Same case. Coronal T$_1$-weighted image

Sellar tubercle meningiomas cause compression in the prefixed chiasm, in the sagittal plane. In postfixed chiasms a hypophyseal adenoma causes compression from below. A postfixed chiasm is compressed from below by craniopharyngiomas and suprasellar epidermoids, and from behind and above by third ventricle gliomas.

Hypophyseal Adenomas

Hypophyseal adenomas, both secreting and inactive, cause endocrinal disorders (Fig. 13). Microadenoma (maximum diameter of 1 cm) is distinguishable by the near normal tissue. It may be expansive (included adenoma) or infiltrative (invasive adenoma).

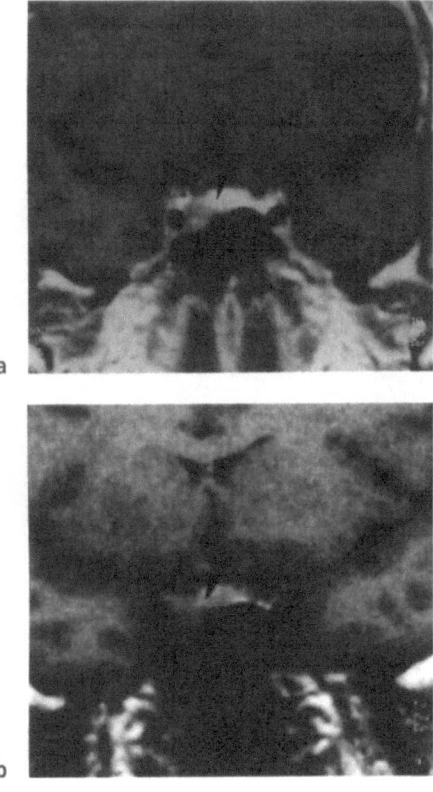

Fig. 13a,b Pituitary microadenoma: 6 mm. **a)** Coronal T_1-weighted image following i.v. contrast enhancement showing hypointense lesions (*arrows*). **b)** Coronal T_1-weighted image, non contrast study (*arrows*)

Prolactinoma is the most frequent adenoma in women. It is characterized by galactorrhea, amenorrhea, gynecomasty, and dyspareunia. *Somatropic adenoma* (GH) leads to gigantism during childhood or to acromegaly in adults.

Adrenocorticotropic hormone (ACTH)-secreting adenoma may be responsible for Cushing's syndrome: ecchymoses, purple striae, hirsutism, emotional lability, and osteoporosis. The compression of the chiasm from below causes superior quadrantic bitemporal hemianopsia.

Craniopharyngioma

The symptomatology of craniopharyngiomas is complex and varied (Fig. 14). In childhood and adolescence cachexia and emaciation are the main signs, whereas in adults psychic disorders and obesity are present.

Visual defects consist of inferior quadrantic bitemporal hemianopsia, which, however, is irregular and asymmetrical.

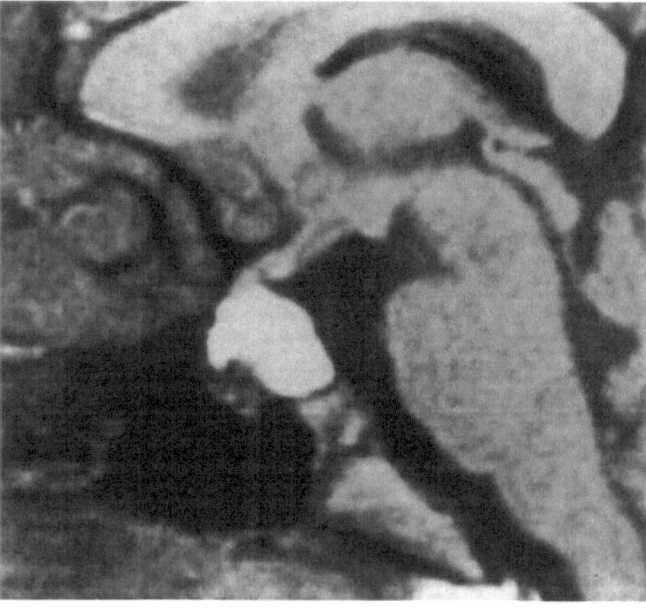

Fig. 14 Calcified craniopharyngioma: 15 mm. Sagittal T$_1$-weighted image demonstrates hyperintensity in the suprasellar region

Early Diagnosis
of Posterior Cranial Fossa Tumors

In relation to the small dimensions of the posterior cranial fossa, a tumor can cause *blockage* of the cerebrospinal fluid and various other symptoms in an early stage. Headache is localized in the suboccipital region with nuchal and neck irradiation or with frontal region irradiation and is often associated with vomiting. In the early stage, vomiting is projectile in character and is not associated with headache. The vomiting occurs mainly in tumors of the fourth ventricle because of the direct compression on the bulbar centers of the vagus.

Tumors of the Cerebellar Vermis

In the initial stage, gait disturbances appear when walking with closed eyes and changing direction; in the late stage these disturbance also become manifest with open eyes, where the gait is uncertain and broad based with a tendency to fall backward – more rarely forward. In a horizontal position the patient can perform movements correctly. Most patients present with pain, rigidity or stiffness of nuchal muscles, and an antalgic posture or stance in flexion or extension.

Tumors of the Cerebellar Hemispheres

Symptoms start with an uncertain gait, homolateral upper limb along the trunk, hypotonia of the muscles of the homolateral limbs with bradykinesia, dysmetria, and adiadochokinesia.

The involvement of the cerebellar peduncles sometimes causes tremor as an early symptom.

Tumors of the Fourth Ventricle

In tumors of the fourth ventricle the first symptom can be vertigo caused by head movements (Fig. 15). The voice can be explosive, marked, and monotonous.

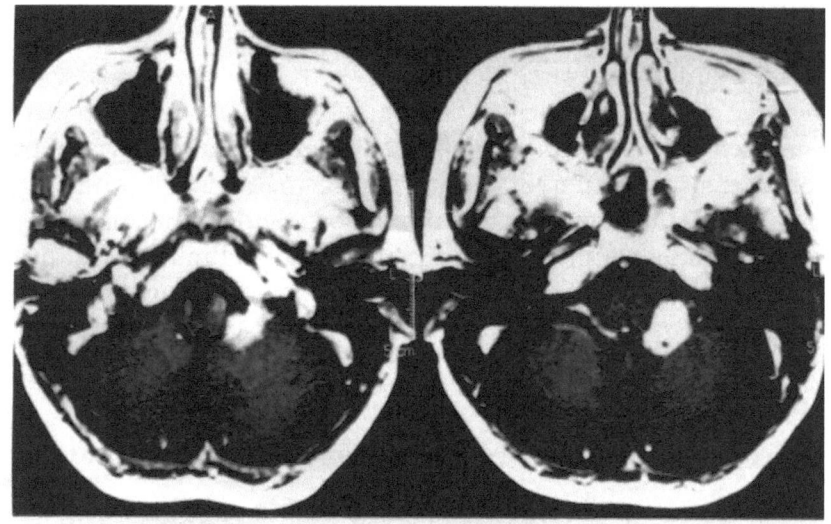

a

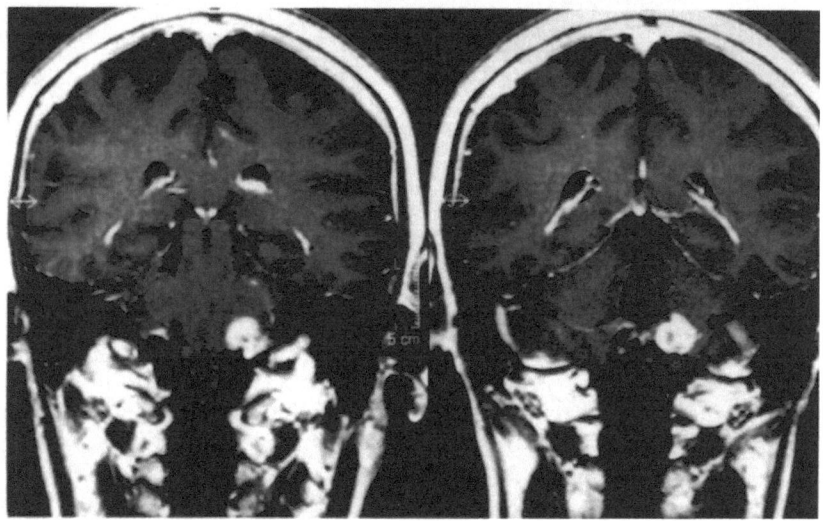

b

Fig. 15a,b Left lateral recess fourth ventricle ependymoma: 15 mm. **a)** Axial T_1-weighted image following i.v. contrast enhancement. **b)** Same case. Coronal T_1-weighted image

Acoustic Neurinomas

Acoustic neurinomas arise from the internal auditory canal and then extend toward the cerebello-pontine angle, less frequently into the labyrinth (Fig. 16).

Intracanalicular acoustic neurinomas are characterized by:
– Unilateral hearing loss
– Tinnitus of high tones
– Dysequilibrium, rarely vertigo

Tone audiogram may demonstrate a unilateral or asymmetrical sensorineural hearing loss; however, hearing may be normal in 5% of small or intracanalicular tumors. Vocal audiogram may detect a decrease in discrimination on the affected side. Brainstem auditory-evoked response (BSAER) is a sensitive test for diagnosing retro-

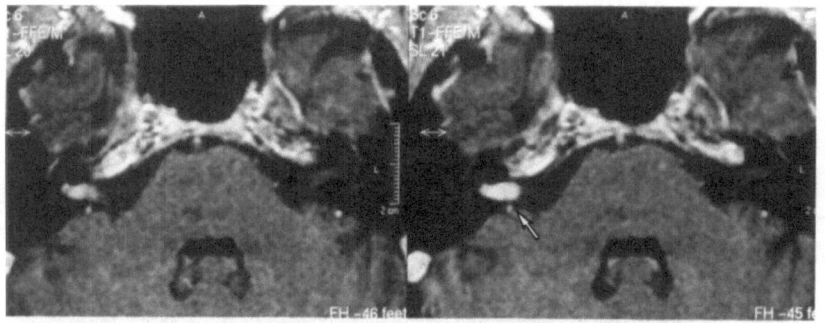

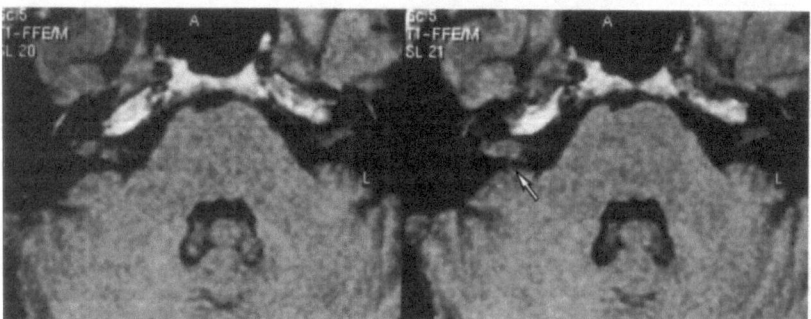

Fig. 16a,b Right intracanalicular VIII n.c. neurinoma: 4 mm. **a)** Axial T_1-weighted image following i.v. contrast enhancement (*arrow*). **b)** Same case; noncontrast study (*arrow*)

choclear pathological conditions and intracanalicular tumors; however, a high rate (33%) of false negatives has been observed because of absence of involvement or compression or ischemia of the tumor on the cochlear nerve.

When the tumors are extracanalicular, trigeminal involvement causes corneal hypoesthesia. A homolateral corneal reflex test should be always performed in cases of suspected hearing loss.
When hypoacusis is present, the absence of the corneal reflex allows early diagnosis even without an instrumental test.

Acoustic Intrameatal Meningioma

Acoustic intrameatal meningiomas are uncommon tumors arising from a small duro-arachnoidal recess situated in the internal auditory canal (Fig. 17). There is no sex prevalence of the tumor but it mainly affects subjects between the fifth and sixth decade of life. Progressive hearing loss is the prevalent symptom, which may be associated with peripheral facial paresis and more rarely with tinnitus. Magnetic resonance imaging (MRI) and computed tomography (CT) scan with bone reconstruction give an excellent topographical definition of micromeningiomas, but a preoperative diagnosis of acoustic intrameatal meningioma is unlikely because there are no radiological findings to distinguish it from vestibular schwanomma, except for indirect signs such as hyperostosis in cases of bone invasion.

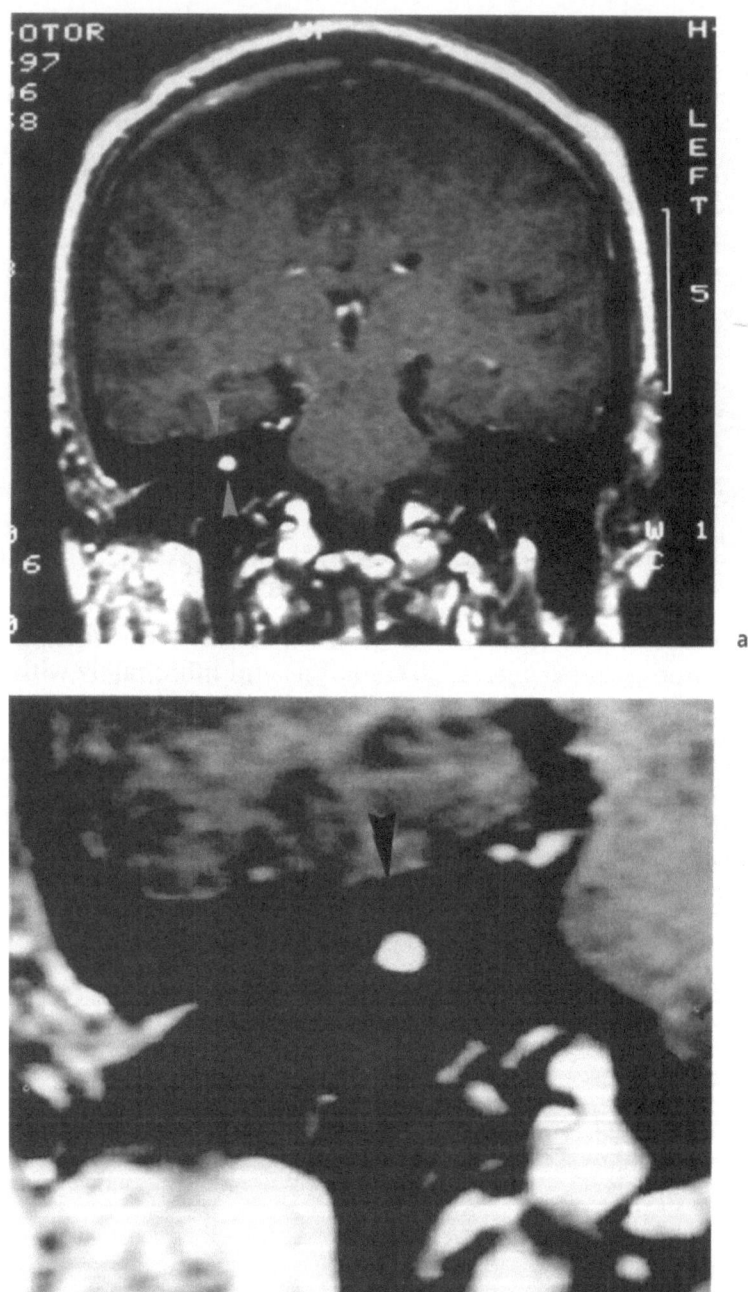

Fig. 17a,b Right intracanalicular meningioma: 4 mm. **a)** Coronal T₁-weighted image following i.v. contrast enhancement (*arrow*). **b)** Enlargement of the same case (*arrow*)

Early Diagnosis
of Spinal Tumors

General Syndrome

Neoplastic spinal lesions make up one of the most important chapters in neurosurgery: the removal of generally benign tumors affecting the spinal cord has represented one of the most advanced and impressive stages in neurological surgery since 1887 when the English surgeon Horsley first removed a spinal tumor following the indications of Gowers, a neurologist who specialized in spinal pathology.

The more frequent causes of spinal cord compression are spinal tumors, degenerative osteoligamentous diseases of the vertebral column, and spinal trauma. Spinal compression, and in particular that caused by spinal tumors, is characterized by its evolution, which is progressive in terms of both time and space. Spinal cord damage therefore can occur either directly through progressive mechanical action at the point of compression or indirectly as the result of a vascular ischemic phenomenon or venous engorgement. What should be underlined is that the lesions are reversible for a long time.

The general syndrome of spinal cord compression is schematically based on pain, weakness, hypoesthesia, and sphinteric disturbances, symptoms which can be divided into two groups:
a) lesional;
b) sublesional, indicating that long tracts are involved.

Lesional symptoms can be represented by: radicular sensory syndrome, radicular motor syndrome, and metameric medullary syndrome, the consequence of damage to the gray matter (anterior and posterior horns) where symptoms and signs are difficult to differentiate from radicular ones. Sublesional symptoms, the consequence of damage to the white matter, cause long-tract medullary syndrome that consists principally of pyramidal, spinothalamic, and posterior funiculi lesions.

Symptoms and Signs

In most spinal tumors the first symptom consists of vertebral, radicular or cordonal pain, followed, in order of frequency, by weakness, sensory disturbances (paresthesia, hypoesthesia), sphincteric and neurovegetative disorders, neurogenic intermittent claudication, and subarachnoid hemorrhage.

Pain

Vertebral Pain or Rachiodynia. Vertebral pain may be the only clinical symptom and is often associated with radicular or cordonal pain. It is perceived as an aching, deep, and indeterminate pain, limited to two or three contiguous vertebral segments, variable in intensity, and perceived in the occipito-cervical, subscapular, dorsal, or lumbar region, often subcontinuously. The pain is exacerbated by vertebral flexion, extension or rotation, and those conditions that increase endorachidial pressure (coughing, sneezing, Valsalva's maneuver); it is usually associated with an antalgic contracture of the paravertebral muscles; and it is short, quickly followed (3-6 months), in most cases, by cordal or radicular weakness, paresthesia, or hypoesthesia.

Radicular Pain. Radicular pain is localized in the dermatomic area of a sensitive root. It is a subcontinuous, gnawing ache, with sudden, sharp spasms that become more serious with intrarachidial hypertension and root traction. This pain is characteristic of an intradural, extramedullary tumor, forming the initial symptom in 60%-70% of cases, whereas it is rarer in extradural (when the tumor involves one or more interpeduncular foramina) and intramedullary tumors (10%-15%, where it is more frequent in lumbosacral gliomas). Radicular pain can also have a medullary origin, i.e., cornual, in relation to posterior horn excitation.

Spinal Cord Pain. In spinal cord tumors the pain is reported as a painful disturbance or a diffuse burning and sometimes as a sudden and sharp spasm which can last some minutes and leave deep, residual pain at the affected site. It is never of radicular distribution but spreads indistinctly in a segment of a limb, in a whole limb, or in more than one limb or in a part, a half, or the whole body.

Cord pain is rare in extradural malignant tumors, although more frequent in intramedullary gliomas, especially bilateral gliomas, than in neurinomas and meningiomas, both at the beginning and, above all, during the evolution of the disease. In intramedullary gliomas, cord pain is more frequent in dorsal and cervical tumors; an important aspect is its slow and progressively descending distribution, never observed in extramedullary tumors.

Motor Deficiency

Motor deficiency is the next most frequent symptom, after pain, and is described as weakness, exhaustion, and numbness of one or more limbs at their distal or proximal extremities; fasciculations are rarely present. Motor disturbances can be due to the damage of one or more anterior roots, to the direct or indirect involvement of the anterior horns (ischemic damage), or to intrinsic or extrinsic compression of the corticospinal tracts. Flaccid motor deficiency results in the first two cases, and spastic in the third, although the two can coexist.

The weakness usually starts from the compression site, in relation to the somatotopic disposition of motor fibers of the cruciate pyramidal tract (after crossing the fibers in the lower limbs they are more external, and those in the upper limbs more internal); the development of motor deficiency is thus ascending in extramedullary and descending in intramedullary tumors, affecting in these the more cranial muscles.

Motor deficiency is rare at the onset of an extradural malignancy and in 2/3 of cases develops into flaccid paralysis. An acute transverse lesion may be present in 20% of cases, including the benign ones. It should also be noted that forms of apoplexy or sudden deterioration, although unusual, are also noted in intramedullary tumors and are caused by sudden edema, or intratumoral hemorrhage or malignant degeneration of the tumor, such as in glioblastomas. Extremely rapid evolution is also described in some cases of extradural meningiomas and is not as rare as might be thought. Developments of this kind are exceptional in neurinomas, however.

Diagnosis was only made in 6% of cases at the onset of weakness as the first symptom. As a rule the weakness in neurinomas, meningiomas, gliomas, and in some extradural malignant or benign tumors has a slow and progressive evolution, sometimes with temporary remissions; this feature is more frequent in vertebral angiomas with medullary compression. The high sensitivity of the pyramidal tract to a direct mechanical action, the great vulnerability of motor cells of the anterior horns to ischemia, and the compression of a motor root explain the high rate (70%) of motor deficiency as a first or second symptom at a relatively early stage.

Paresthesia

Like pain, motor deficiencies, and hypoesthesia, paresthesia can have radicular (or cornual) and cordonal, uni- or bilateral distribution. Paresthesias are persistent sensations perceived, without a triggering event, as sensations of tingling, pricking, numbness, or heat and cold. They spread over the thorax, abdomen, and along one or more limbs. As an isolated initial symptom, paresthesia is unusual: 7%-9%.

In meningiomas the sensations constitute, after pain, the most frequent initial symptom (27-37%) and are mainly in the spinal cord, of distal origin. They show ascending progression in extramedullary tumors and descending progression in intramedullary ones. In gliomas the progression can be irregular.

Sensory Deficiency

A spinal tumor rarely presents with symptoms of sensory deficiency. A reduction of sensory discrimination, "dead skin" sensitivty, or the loss of feeling in a finger, a limb or a part of it, are considered sensory deficiencies. They can consist of hypoesthesia or anesthesia and may involve deep and/or surface sensitivity, sometimes with tabetic and syringomyelic features. They can be metameric, due to cornual or radicular involvement (2% of cases in the precocious stage), present at a superior level, or be suspended as in the case of cord compromise (3.6% of cases in the initial stage).

The disposition of fibers in the spinothalamic tract explains the first extension to the distal dermatomes and the descent in the intramedullary ones, with, in the latter case, damage to the dermatomes closest to the tumor.

It should be underlined that metameric hypoanesthesia is more frequent in the early phases and, for a final diagnosis, must be searched for in the patient history because further progression may conceal it; metameric hypoanesthesia constitutes the most important, if not pathognomonic, sign of an intramedullary lesion; it has seldom been noticed in extramedullary compression, but less rarely in spondylogenetic myelopathy. Cordal anesthesia was the first symptom in 6% of intradural extramedullary benign tumors but has never been found in intramedullary and extradural tumors as the first symptom.

Sphinteric Disturbances

Sphinteric disturbances are rare as the initial symptom in either extramedullary or intramedullary benign tumors. In conus medullaris tumors they are common at the start of clinical history.

Sexual Disturbances

Impotentia erigendi and impotentia coeundi are very unusual as initial symptoms. They are also unusual as the initial symptom in conus medullaris tumors.

Subarachnoid Hemorrhage

Subarachnoid hemorrhage secondary to a spinal tumor is a classic but very rare event in neurosurgery. The patient feels a sharp dorsal or dorsolumbar pain (in conocaudal tumours), without loss of consciousness.

A meningeal syndrome can be established and is associated, in cono-caudal gliomas, with cruralgia and sciatalgia; the cerebrospinal fluid is blood-stained. It can be spontaneous or caused by a trauma or strong exertion. It is present more often in conocaudal ependymomas.

The tumor histology is of considerable importance here: the filum terminale of ependymomas has a loose, highly vascular connectival texture, unlike dense and resistant connectival-capsulated ependymomas at other levels. The frequency at the conus and caudal levels also has another explanation: here the mechanical stresses are greater during neck and rachis movements, and, indeed, in one out of three cases the hemorrhage occurs during physical activity.

Neurogenic Intermittent Claudication

Intermittent claudication is a typical symptom of medullary stress. It consists of weakness and hyposthenia first in one lower limb, then in the other, which develops while walking and decreases after a few minutes' rest; it starts again when walking is resumed. Functional restoration becomes subsequently incomplete and spastic parasparesis occurs. During the initial phase, neurologic examination is negative when the patient is at rest, while first hypertonia and an increase of deep reflexes, then evident pyramidal signs are revealed when under stress. Sensitivity remains intact and sphincteric disturbances are rare at the beginning. It can be present in lumbar canal stenosis and in vascular malformations.

Transverse Section Syndrome

Vertebral angioma can reveal itself in this manner, at times following a trauma or pregnancy. Hemorrhagic tumors can also start with this syndrome.

The Early Syndrome

The need to associate the *first symptom* with the subsequent one becomes clear when we consider that spinal tumors present through pain in 70% of cases and with paresthesia and hypoesthesia in 5%-20%, complaints usually attributable to several diseases such as "arthritis", "neuritis", or "visceral diseases". The *second symptom* is almost always diagnostically clearer and defines or contributes to determining an organic neurological syndrome with features of a medullary, radicular, or radiculomedullary lesion, hence, the utility of studying it. The second symptom is, in fact, well remembered by patients because it is more serious than the first one.

The frequency, association, and type of complaint vary according to the site of the tumor; it is thus essential to examine the early syndrome in relation to it.

Cervical Tumors

More than 50% of cervical tumors are neurinomas and meningiomas, followed by intramedullary tumors (30%) and extradural malignancies (6%-7%).

Neurinomas frequently arise from nerve roots IV-V-VI, whereas meningiomas primarily affect the higher cervical segments; at the foramen magnum the meningioma/neurinoma relation is 6:1. In childhood and adolescence there is a greater incidence of glioma (in particular astrocytomas, seldom ependymomas). The most schematic early syndrome is seen in *neurinomas*: unilateral, monoradicular, persistent pain often occurring at night, increased by decubitus, and followed after some time by various degrees of hypoesthesia or weakness at the same radicular level. This is almost pathognomonic in neurinomas, although such pain can also be caused by lateral disc herniation, but in the latter condition the pain is sharper and the onset and development of weakness faster.

More frequently *meningiomas* cause a short initial syndrome comprising above all paresthesia and radicular pain, and sometimes unilateral weakness, followed by early motor and/or sensitive long-tract involvement.

In foramen magnum tumors, more often meningiomas, the initial complaint, affect the upper limbs in particular. In foramen magnum meningiomas and neurinomas, the early syndrome is almost the same and is characterized by an often strong occipital pain, followed by paresthesias and/or paresis in one upper limb or both, in contrast with the rule whereby cervical neurinomas and meningiomas never, in the initial stage of the disease, affect the upper limbs (except for radicular deficiency) but rather involve the homolateral lower limb and then the contralateral one.

In this very early stage, beyond the syndromes that are characteristic of neurinoma or meningioma, and sometimes within their fields, X-rays can frequently provide the diagnosis: enlargement of a neural foramen almost always indicates a neurinoma.

The onset of *extradural malignancy* is characterized by a sharp radicular pain (50% of cases), often pluriradicular, alone or with tenacious vertebral pain or radicular paresthesia. Uni- or bilateral weakness develops rapidly, starting or immediately appearing as more severe in the lower limbs.

In *intramedullary tumors* only radicular pain, uni- or bilaterally, is rare, both at the beginning and at the late stages of the disease; the pain is indicative only when it clearly possesses the features of cornual pain. Cordal pain has an important diagnostic value when localized in the trunk and/or in the lower limbs, but rarely occurs. Actually, even without this pain, weakness is present in more than 70% of cases as a primary or secondary symptom and can have great diagnostic value. In most cases radicular paresis is limited to the upper limbs (bilaterally from the beginning or subsequently affecting the limbs), sometimes preceded by fasciculations and linked to the paresthesias or to a uni- or bilateral touch and temperature hypoesthesia. These disturbances are due to involvement of the anterior and posterior horns and the spinothalamic tract. In our patients with astrocytomas and other gliomas the weakness arose earlier and was more frequent than in ependymomas.

Cervico-dorsal gliomas, those with simultaneous involvement of contiguous cervical and dorsal segments, can cause an early syndrome with features different from those of dorsal or cervical gliomas. Vertebral pain can simultaneously involve the nape of the neck and the back. The weakness can be serious or only moderately spastic or paraparetic but associated with hypotrophy of the small hand muscles. This syndrome is common in cervical spondylotic myelopathy, which can cause segmental hypoesthesia with vascular pathogenesis, although here the pseudomyotonic phenomenon of hand opening is common, if not pathognomonic, and characterized by a remarkable slowness in the extension motion of the first, and especially in the fourth and fifth finger, while closing the fingers is strong and fast. The weakness in the extension of the fingers has to be accompanied by a remarkable pyramidalization of the hand. This motor syndrome of the small hand muscle can be caused by anterior or midline meningiomas, not infrequently with fasciculations, and by some inferior cervical neurinomas as a result of involvement of the anterior spinal artery.

Dorsal Tumors

The dorsal region is the most frequent location of neoplastic compressions of the spinal cord (Figs. 19, 20).

About 40%-51% of *neurinomas* are found here, with a male preponderance (3:2). In neurinomas radicular pain is the most frequent initial symptom, but the diagnosis is made later than for cervical neurinoma because radicular pain can reproduce a visceral pain. In fact, in most cases the early syndrome is marked by initial monoradicular pain, uni- or bilaterally, combined with motor long-tract signs. Of spinal *meningiomas* 70%-85% arise in the dorsal column. The female/male ratio is 4:1; in children, rare meningiomas occurred in girls more often. In dorsal meningiomas the initial stage is mono- and oligosymtomatic, with radicular and vertebral pain, sometimes combined with long-tract sensory or motor deficiency, and, above all, paresthesias at the distal end of the lower limbs.

There is a high incidence (60%) of *extradural malignancies*, especially those with metastasis. In childhood, primitive tumors are more frequent: sarcomas usually in children around the age of 10

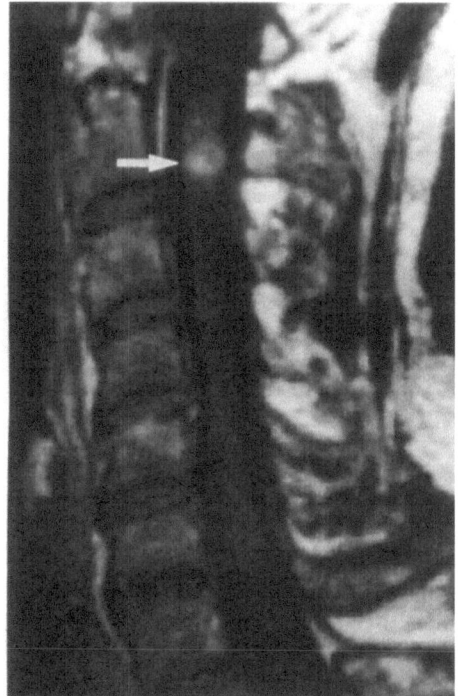

a

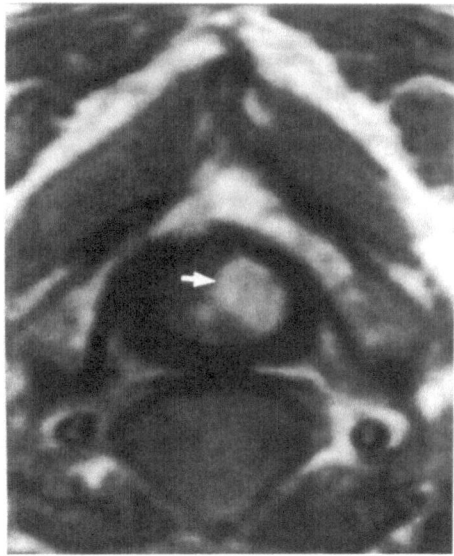

b

Fig. 19a,b a) Astrocytoma C_2: 12 mm. Sagittal T_1-weighted image following i.v. contrast enhancement (*arrow*). **b)** Same case. Axial T_1-weighted image following i.v. contrast enhancement showing right intramedullary location (*arrow*)

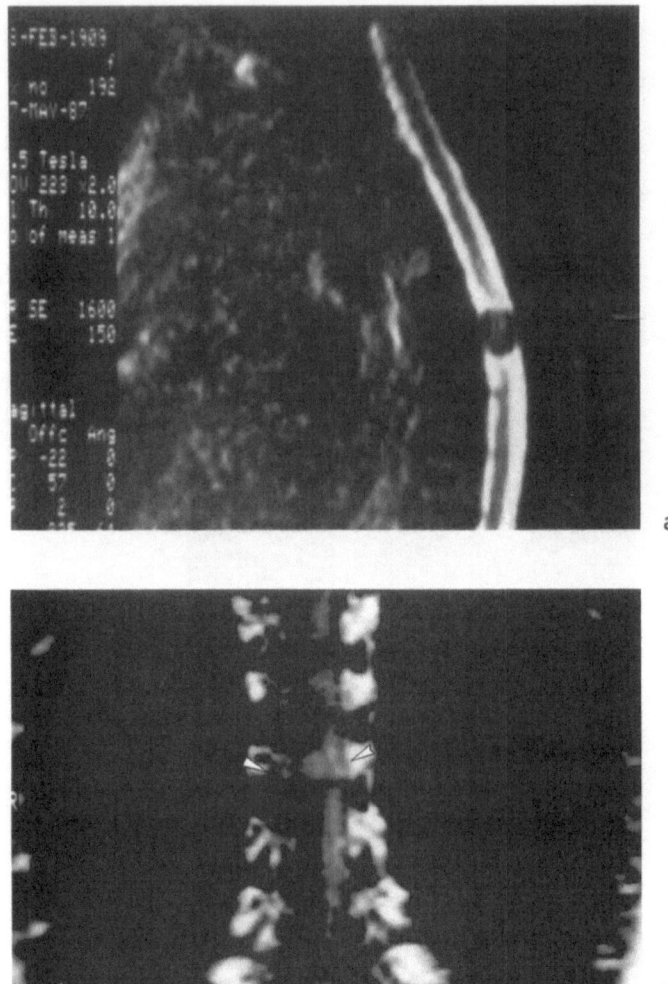

Fig. 20a,b Meningioma D_6: 15 mm. **a)** Sagittal T_2-weighted image showing hypointense lesion dislocating spinal cord. **b)** Coronal T_1-weighted image following i.v. contrast enhancement. The lesion dislocated the spinal cord on the left (*arrows*)

and sympatoblastomas (neuroblastomas) in those aged 0-3. The Brown-Sequard syndrome does not always correspond to that reported for cervical localization: severe vertebral pain (60%), but also radicular pain (24%), at times combined; subacute evolution of medullary compression with sensory and motor deficiency, distally at first, and moderate increase of ESR.

Radicular pain, especially pluriradicular, is severe, often bilateral, "belt like," and has great diagnostic value. The evolution is more rapid than in cervical compressions not only becuase the dorsal canal is narrow, but above all because of the high rate of metastases (60%), which develop faster than primary tumors, and the greater vulnerability of dorsal cord circulation. The onset of weakness in the lower limbs in most cases not only manifests itself abruptly but, contrary to cervical localizations, rapidly evolves into paraplegia. Although rare, apoplectic onset and rapid evolution have also been noted in other spinal tumors.

Dorsal and lumbosacral *gliomas* show a different frequency (39%-58%). The early syndrome is characterized by a frequently painful mono- or paraparesis. more often cordal or vertebral than radicular, with or without sensory impairment, and rarely with sphinteric disturbances. We have to stress that, in our patients with gliomas, a motor impairment, unilateral at first, has never become bilateral during the early stage of the disease. When it was bilateral, it arose or developed with this feature.

At an early stage, initial radicular pain thus suggests a neurinoma; more rarely, it indicates a meningioma and, sporadically, a glioma.

A clinical aspect frequently encountered in the early stage of dorsal gliomas is cordal pain localized in the thorax and abdomen with descending evolution; the most important and constant sign is segmental hypo-anesthesia. Dorsal fasciculation can be observed.

Lumbosacral gliomas often begin with radicular pain, and in most cases are mistaken for sciatic pain secondary to disc herniation.

Tumoral sciatic pain is difficult to interpret when no other complaints are present. The intermittent pain, typical of disc herniation, is often observed in oncogenic sciatalgias. Exacerbation of pain at night, together with a negative result of the straight-leg-raising test, are the most indicative signs of a spinal tumor. As mentioned above, neoplastic sciatic pain is always attributed to disc herniation, the misunderstanding stemming from epidemiological criteria: the incidence of disc herniation is far higher than that of spinal tumors.

In lumbosacral gliomas the sciatic pain is not as clear as in neurinomas and often involves cornual pain, which is lacerating and burning; it can last for a considerable length of time as an initial symptom and may suggest an intramedullary tumor when the first and second motor neuron are involved, sometimes with fasciculation and irregular hypoesthesia.

Cono-filum Tumors

Given that the spinal canal is very wide at the lumbosacral level, that the lumbar enlargement corresponds to D10-D11-D12-L1, and that under L1 there are lumbar, sacral, and coccygeal roots (cauda equina), a small D12-L1 tumor can affect a number of neuromeres and even more roots. Moreover, a caudal tumor can reach a remarkable size before clinical manifestations arise. If the compression is at the epiconus or caudal level, the impairment will be different, spastic paraparesis and sensory deficiency with a level, and flaccid paresis with sensory radicular deficiency respectively.

Meningioma. Lumbar meningiomas are rare. Radicular pain is often the first symptom and, if exacerbated by column motion or decubitus, can be long-lasting. It can spread as sciatica, uni- or, more rarely, bilaterally, vertebral pain indicating the segment of one of the affected roots.

Sensory Deficiency. "Saddle" and perianal or genital hypoanesthesia are the main sensory deficiencies provoked by tumors affecting the third, fourth, fifth sacral root or the corresponding neuromeres.

Motor Deficiency. Spastic or flaccid paresis or paralysis can be observed. In the early stages, fasciculations without evident atrophy can be observed but weakness and hypotonia are already present; the preservation of anal and bulbocavernous reflex indicates integrity of the conus.

Sexual and Sphincteric Disorders. When the conus is involved, urgent micturition and incontinence develop soon. Later on, constipation and fecal incontinence become evident.

Neurinoma. Neurinoma can begin with sciatic pain (whereas it is rare in meningiomas), although it is more frequently associated with either spastic-flaccid motor deficiency or radicular-cordal sensory deficiency with regular distribution (whereas in gliomas it is irregular). This also occurs when the initial disturbance is abdominoinguinal neuralgia or lumbocruralgia; it is more frequent in neurinomas but not uncommon in gliomas (Fig. 21).

Extradural Malignancy. Extradural malignant tumors can start with serious vertebral pains, often combined with violent and widespread radicular pain in the lower limbs. This pain is rapidly followed by serious uni- or bilateral flaccid and spastic-flaccid motor deficiency.

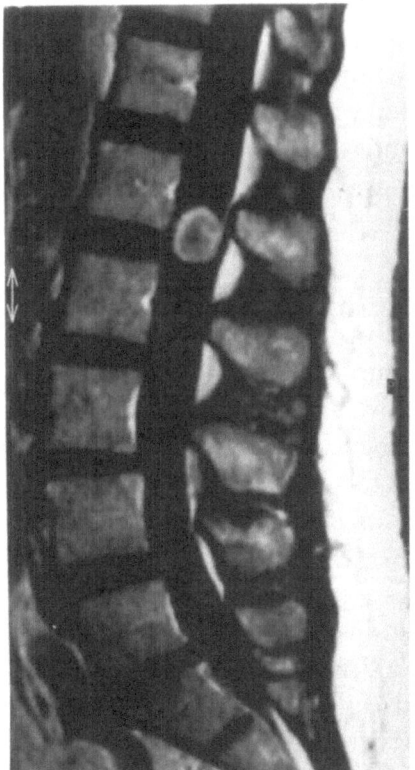 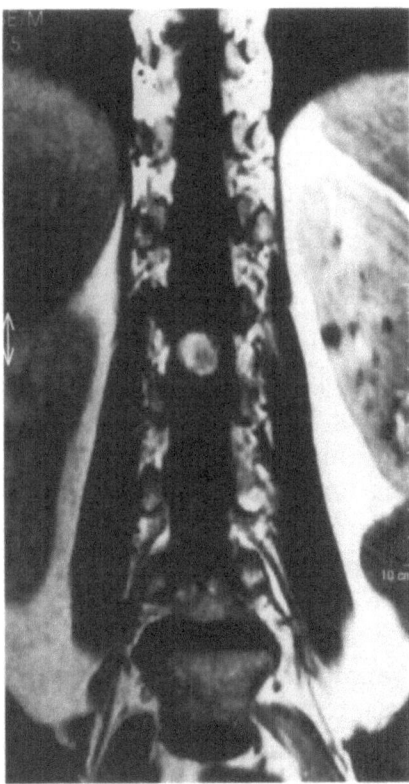

a   b

Fig. 21a,b Neurinoma L_1: 10 mm. **a)** Sagittal T_1-weighted image following i.v. contrast enhancement. **b)** Same cases. Coronal T_1-weighted image

Pathological Anatomy

Spinal tumors can be divided into intradural and extradural, intradural into intra- and extramedullary.

Intradural Extramedullary Tumors

In most cases intradural extramedullary tumors consist of meningiomas, neurinomas, and neurofibromas. Dysembryogenetic tumors (dermoid, epidermoid and neurenteric cysts), or malignant neoplasias (metastasis of hematic and CSF origin) are rare.

Meningioma. Meningiomas are benign tumors with a clear predominance in women, with the greatest incidence between the fifth and seventh decade. They comprise nearly 25% of spinal tumors and nearly 13% of all meningiomas. Spinal meningioma is more frequent at the dorsal segment. It originates in the arachnoid cells and consists of a firm mass, more frequently anterolateral to the spinal cord. Dural attachment of the lesion is always present. The most common histological type at spinal level is the transitional, psammomatous meningioma.

Neurinoma. Together with neurofibroma, this constitutes 25%-30% of intradural extramedullary tumors. A neurinoma, or schwannoma, consists of an encapsulated, ovalar, lobulated, whitish mass. The radicular structures appear eccentric to the mass, running into the tumor capsule. Histologically it is formed by interwoven bundles of spindle cells (Type A of Antoni) or by a looser, mixoid texture (Type B of Antoni).

Neurofibroma. Frequently observed in von Recklinghausen's neurofibromatosis, a neurofibroma has a firmer texture than a neurinoma, is less clearly demarcated, and cannot be dissected from the roots that run through the tumor. Microscopically it is composed of Schwann's cells, fibroblasts, and collagen fibers intermingled in a mucoid or mixoid matrix.

Dermoid Cysts. Dermoid cysts constitute 0.5%-1% of spinal tumors, but reach a rate of 10% in childhood. They are congenital lesions that more frequently develop in the lumbar segment. Musculoskeletal anomalies such as spina bifida or dermal sinus are frequently present. They appear as different-sized, well demarcated, opaque, ovalar masses. The cut surface reveals a yellowish, butter-like material.

Epidermoid Cysts. Epidermoid cysts are rarer than dermoid cysts. Macroscopically they appear as small pearly masses with a butter-like content, rich in cholesterol.

Extradural Tumors

These derive from osteoligamentous and condroid structures of the spinal column with subsequent involvement of the nervous structures.

Benign Bone Tumors

Osteoid Osteoma. Osteoid osteomas constitute nearly 12% of primitive bone tumors at all sites and 6% of spinal bone tumors. They appear as a small, brownish, well-demarcated mass, 1-2 cm in diameter.

Osteoblastoma. Rarer than osteoid osteomas, osteoblastomas represent nearly 1% of bone tumors. They are classified together with osteoid osteomas, the difference between them being represented by the size of the lesion: lesions under 2 cm in diameter are defined as osteoid osteomas, while larger tumors are osteoblastomas.

Giant-Cell Tumors. Giant-cell tumors account for nearly 5% of primitive bone tumors. The incidence in the vertebral column is 2%-5%. There is a slight predominance in women, with a greater incidence occurring roughly in the third decade. The tumor is seen more frequently at the sacral level, in most cases involving the verte-bral body.

Malignant Bone Tumors

Osteosarcoma. After metastatic lesions, osteosarcomas are the most common malignant bone tumors. They affect fast-growing bones and thus are more easily noticed in long-bone metaphysis or in pathological conditions of fast bone rearrangement, such as Paget's disease, or during radiotherapy. They are commonly associated with bilateral retinoblastoma. Macroscopically they appear as a highly vascularized mass composed of an osseous neoformation in various phases of calcification.

Ewing's Sarcoma. At the spinal level Ewing's sarcomas are very rare, constituting 0.5% of malignant bone tumors of the column, with a definite predominance in men above all during the first two decades of life.

Cartilaginous Tumors

Osteochondroma. Although a rather frequent bone tumor (8%-9% of all bone tumors), osteochondromas are rare at the spinal level (1%-4%). They are benign and generally solitary but multiple in 10% of cases. Macroscopically the tumor consists of a small exostotic mass arising from spinous apophyses or from transverse processes.

Chondrosarcoma. Chondrosarcomas are malignant tumors which form in chondroid tissue both as a degeneration of a benign cartilaginous tumor (secondary chondrosarcoma) in 15% of cases, and as a primary malignant one in 85%.

Lipoma. Lipomas are classified among the congenital malformations of spinal occult dysraphism and are associated with meningocele, dermic sinus, and tethered cord.

Angiolipoma. A benign tumor which comprises 0.1%-1.2% of spinal tumors, angiolipomas are more commonly extradural, even if some sporadic intramedullary cases have been reported.

Chordoma. About 1000 cases of chordoma have been reported in the literature. Forming about 18% of malignant bone tumors, they have an ectodermic (notochordal) origin. In spite of its embryologic origin, the tumor does not, in spinal chordoma, appear in the nucleous pulposus but rather in the vertebral body, probably as a result of notochordal tissue at this level.

Vascular Bone Tumors

Vertebral Angioma. While not rare (10%-12% in autoptic series), vertebral angiomas can be symptomatic in about 1% of cases, with a clear predominance in women. It is a slow-growing tumor composed of pathological vessels characterized by endothelial cells spread into a stroma formed by bone trabeculae and fat tissue.

Aneurysmal Bone Cyst. An aneurysmal bone cyst consists of a highly vascularized, multiloculated, osteolytic lesion.

Spinal Metastases

Spinal metastasesare (Fig. 22) the most common malignant lesions of the column, autoptic series revealing vertebral metastases in 15%-40% of patients who died as a result of disseminated neoplasms. All vertebral bodies can be affected, although the low dorsal and lumbar tracts are more frequently involved. In adults, metastases from lung, breast, and prostatic carcinoma are frequent.

Intramedullary Tumors

Intramedullary tumors derive mainly from glial medullary cells and vascular structures and are rarely metastatic lesions.

Glial Tumors

Ependymomas, astryrocytomas, and, rarely, glioblastoma multiforme are glial tumors.

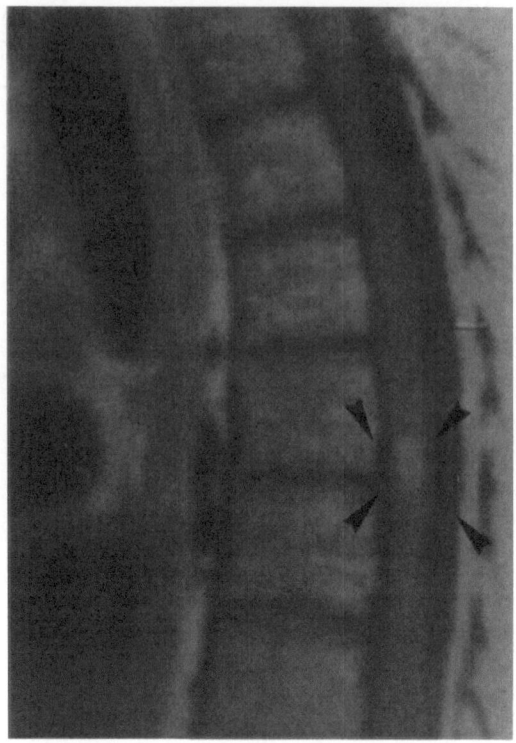

Fig. 22 Spinal metastasis at D_6-D_7 level: 8 mm. Sagittal T_1-weighted image following i.v. contrast enhancement (*arrows*)

Ependymoma. Ependymomas constitute 4%-6% of CNS tumors, about 1/3 of which affect the spinal cord, representing the most frequent intramedullary tumor in adults.

Macroscopically the spinal cord appears enlarged, the vessel stretched and distended. The tumor often appears demarcated, with a well-defined cleavage plane, and intra- or peritumoral cysts are usually present. Histologically they are benign, originating from ependyma cells, mostly in the posterior part of the spinal cord, among the posterior cords, and can affect a number of spinal metameres. They can be removed totally. Some originate from the filum terminale or conofilum causing a cono-caudal compression syndrome.

Astrocytoma. In adulthood astrocytomas represent 30%-40% of intramedullary tumors and about 70% in childhood. The spinal cord is affected by macroscopic morphologic modifications similar to those found in ependymoma, except for the delimitation of the surrounding parenchyma, which appears fully infiltrated by the tumor, and without a clear-cut cleavage plane. This makes the total removal of the mass possible, though not easy. Histologically they are usually fibrillary astrocytomas.

Glioblastoma Multiforme. Glioblastoma multiforme is quite rare and forms 0.2%-1.5% of intramedullary tumors, the literature reporting some 200 cases. It is infiltrative, friable, variegated. Histologically it is characterized by a remarkable cellular polymorphism, with necrosis and vascular proliferation areas with frequent, atypical mitosis.

Vascular Structure Tumors

Hemangioblastoma. Accounting for 1.5% of intramedullary tumors, hemangioblastomas are spheroid, highly vascularized, and often cystic.

Spinal Cavernous Angioma. The incidence of spinal cavernous angioma accounts for some 0.1-0.5% of spinal tumors. Macroscopically and histologically it resembles cerebral cavernoma. The tumor appears as a small reddish-brown mass that can be removed totally.

Intramedullary Metastases

Intramedullary metastases are very rare and can be of hematic or CSF origin (Fig. 22).

Radiological Aspects

MRI is the method of choice for studying these neoplasias and is better than CT in identifying small tumors. However, it is difficult to establish the malignant grade of astrocytomas with MRI.

Glioblastoma Multiforme

Glioblastoma is not observed by a physician until a late stage. Therefore, the concept of an "early diagnosis" is relative. If this tumor arises in cortical epileptogenic areas, seizures develop and an early neuroradiological diagnosis can be established.

On MRI glioblastoma appears as an irregularly roundish mass. In spite of its invasive nature this tumor is well circumscribed. It is surrounded by edema that, in an early stage, may only be mild. Usually, this tumor appears inhomogeneously hypointense on T1-weighted and hyperintense on T2-weighted MRI images with a central and marked hyperintense component due to frequently necrotic degenerative phenomena. After paramagnetic contrast medium administration, a marked and inhomogeneous peripheral enhancement is usually present. In these cases, differential diagnosis must consider metastases. These frequently involve the junction between white and gray matter and are often multiple. Finally, differential diagnosis is from cerebral abscess, mainly if the peripheral component of the tumor is not well circumscribed and is regular. In this case, perfusion-weighted MRI is helpful in demonstrating pathological vascularization of the tumor that presents a perfusion rate higher than in normal cerebral parenchyma. The abscess inside appears as a hypoperfused mass on MRI.

Anaplastic Astrocytoma

An early diagnosis of anaplastic astrocytoma can be made more frequently than for glioblastoma. On MRI anaplastic astrocytoma appears as an inhomogeneous hypointense area on T2-weighted and inhomogeneous hyperintense area on T2-weighted images, with irregular, not well circumscribed margins; it is difficult to establish the border between the tumor and the perilesional edema. Rarely, hemorrhagic nuclei are present. Usually there are no necrotic-cystic or calcified areas. Contrast enhancement is absent or slightly inhomogeneous.

Astrocytoma

Astrocytomas are characterized by homogeneous signal intensity, hypointense on T1-weighted and hyperintense on T2-weighted MRI images. Occasionally, inhomogeneous signals are found. These radiological features are due to the histological type of the tumor. It consists of well-differentiated neoplastic and normal astrocytes. Because of the slow growth of this tumor, perilesional edema does not form. There is no contrast enhancement because newly formed vessels are absent. Sometimes differential diagnosis with cerebral ischemia is difficult, mainly if the tumor shows a superficial extension, causing a cortical thickening. In these cases the different localization and the non ictal onset of the tumor can be helpful. If the diagnosis is doubtful, the study of cerebral perfusion by MRI can distinguish this tumor because it shows increased perfusion in the tumor and decreased perfusion in the ischemic area.

Pilocytic Astrocytoma

Pilocytic astrocytoma is the most common astrocytoma in the pediatric age group. Early diagnosis is important because total surgical excision is thought to be curative in nearly 100% of cases, without adjuvant therapy. Pilocytic astrocytoma is often associated with neurofibromatosis, especially if it is located in anterior optic pathways.

On MRI the tumor appears as a well-circumscribed mass with a roundish or multilobular morphology. This tumor often has a mural nodule and a cystic component which appears hypointense on T1-weighted and hyperintense on T2-weighted images, whereas the solid component shows an intensity similar to that of the gray matter because of its hypercellularity. After intravenous administration of contrast medium the lesion presents a marked and homogeneous enhancement because of the richly vascularized tumor. Usually there is no peritumoral edema or calcification. Although pilocytic astrocytomas show characteristic radiological features, differential diagnosis from ganglioglioma and pleomorphic xanthoastrocytoma must be kept in mind, especially in superficial cerebral hemispheric localizations.

Central Neurocytoma

Central neurocytomas are tumors of subependymal origin and considered to be benign. They usually develop in the region of the foramen of Monro and protrude into the supratentorial ventricular area. On MRI a central neurocytoma appears as a mass extending into the lateral ventricles, with a roundish morphology and inhomogeneous signal on both T1- and T2-weighted images. The signal is due to the presence of calcifications. A marked contrast enhancement is present because the tumor is highly vascularized.

Oligodendroglioma

On CT and MRI the appearance of oligodendroglioma is characteristic: it is localized in the frontal or fronto-temporal cortex, calcifications can be observed in 90% of cases, and sometimes the tumor is associated with cranial thecal alterations. Cystic components and calcifications are frequent and are distinctly seen on MRI. Edema is mild or absent. Oligodendrogliomas have an inhomogeneous signal; it is seen as a hypointense area with hyperintense nuclei on T1-weighted and as hyperintense with hypointense nuclei on T2-weighted images. A slight contrast enhancement is observed in 50% of cases.

Ganglioglioma and Gangliocytoma

Ganglioglioma is a mixed tumor, formed by neuronal and glial cells. It affects primarily children and young adults and mainly develops in a supratentorial location, especially temporal.

Gangliocytomas are rarer than gangliogliomas. They are formed predominantly by differentiated neuronal components and scarce glial ones. Both histologically and radiologically the differential diagnosis between ganglioglioma and gangliocytoma is difficult.

The slow growth and frequent onset of seizures allow an early diagnosis at a time when surgical excision is possible.

On MRI these tumors appear as well-circumscribed solid masses. Gangliogliomas can present calcifications. The signal characteristics are not specific. They are hypointense on T1-weighted and hyperintense with inhomogeneous areas on T2-weighted images. Gradient echo sequences or CT are suggested for determining the presence of calcifications. Differential diagnosis is between these tumors and pilocytic astrocytomas, but the latter are more commonly found in deep sites and do not have calcifications.

Astrocytoma of the Cerebellum

Astrocytoma of the cerebellum is the most frequent tumor in children, the peak of incidence being in the second decade of life. The postoperative survival is very long (94% of cases - 25-year survival).

Pilocytic astrocytoma is one of the more common astrocytomas of the cerebellum.

These tumors present morphological and radiological characteristics similar to those of supratentorial astrocytomas (see above) and are often associated with neurofibromatosis.

MRI is the method of choice for identifying this tumor. Using this technique cerebellar astrocytomas appear as a well-delimited, roundish mass, often with a cystic component and a richly vascularized mural nodule. The cystic component appears hypointense on T1-weighted and homogeneously hyperintense on T2-weighted MRI images. The mural nodule appears isointense on T1-weighted images compared with the cerebral cortex and isointense on T2-weighted images compared with the cerebral cortex because of its high cellularity.

After intravenous administration of a paramagnetic contrast medium marked enhancement of the wall and mural nodule is present. This is due to rich vascularization of these components. Perilesional edema, if present, is scarce. Rarely some calcifications are found.

Medulloblastoma

Medulloblastoma is one of the more common pediatric brain tumors and the most frequently found primitive neuroectodermal tumor (PNET). This term defines a wide group of tumors such as ependymoblastoma, neuroblastoma, and pineoblastoma.

Medulloblastomas often arise in the cerebellar vermis and cause an early triventricular hydrocephalus due to compression of the fourth ventricle. Localizations in the cerebellar hemisphere are found less frequently than in the cerebellar vermis and invade the ponto-cerebellar angle. On MRI medulloblastoma has a rather characteristic appearance as a median or paramedian mass localized behind the fourth ventricle with associated hydrocephalus; it is hyperintense on T2-weighted images and isointense with respect to the gray matter. Hydrocephalus is often present. At times, inhomogeneous signals can be present because of intratumoral hemorrhage and necrotic components.

Ependymoma

Ependymomas are seen more frequently during childhood, the peak incidence being between 10 and 15 years. They comprise 10% of pediatric brain tumors. Ependymomas arise from the ependyma coating the ventricles; the floor of the fourth ventricle is the site of predilection. They tend to occupy the fourth ventricle, causing early triventricular hydrocephalus. On MRI this tumor appears as an intraventricular mass with an inhomogeneous signal due to cystic areas, necrosis, calcifications and hemorrhage. Hydrocephalus is often present. Calcifications are present in 45% of cases and make it possible to distinguish ependymomas from medulloblastomas. They are easily seen on gradient echo sequences and on CT. Contrast enhancement is always present.

Hemangioblastoma

Hemangioblastomas are benign tumors, constituting about 7% of the posterior cranial fossa tumors in adults. They are often associated with Hippel-Lindau disease. Cerebellar hemisphere and vermis are the sites most often involved. Hemangioblastomas can sometimes be present in the brainstem but rarely in the spinal cord. The supratentorial localization is exceptional. Usually, this tumor is solitary, but multiple lesions can be found when associated with von Hippel-Lindau disease or located in the spine.

On MRI hemangioblastomas appear as a roundish mass with a cystic component and a vascularized mural nodule.

The mural nodule shows a slightly increased signal intensity compared to that of the cerebral cortex.

Characteristic signs, thought to be pathognomonic by some authors, are pathological vascular structures with a serpentine morphology. These findings are important in the differential diagnosis and are often detected by MRI, though rarely by CT.

Meningioma

On MRI meningiomas appear as an isointense mass compared to the cerebral parenchyma on T1-weighted and hyperintense on proton density- (PD) and T2-weighted images. In these latter sequences meningiomas present, in 50% of cases, a signal intensity similar to that of the cerebral cortex; in 35% of cases it appears slightly hyperintense and in 15% of cases hypointense. Most meningiomas present a variable grade of signal heterogeneity on T2-weighted images due to: calcifications, cystic components, and tumoral vascularization. Paramagnetic contrast medium administration allows a clear definition of tumoral borders and relations to nearby structures. The probable infiltration of the meningeal surface adjacent to the tumor is another important piece of information given by contrast-enhanced MRI. In about 1/3 of cases, histological study demonstrates a meningeal thickening and infiltration that can extend some centimeters from the tumor. In these cases, the infiltrated dura, "dural tail," can be visualized on contrast-enhanced MRI (Fig. 18).

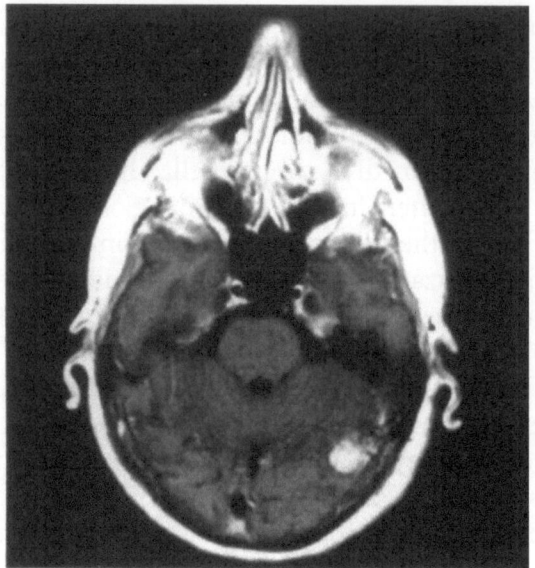

a

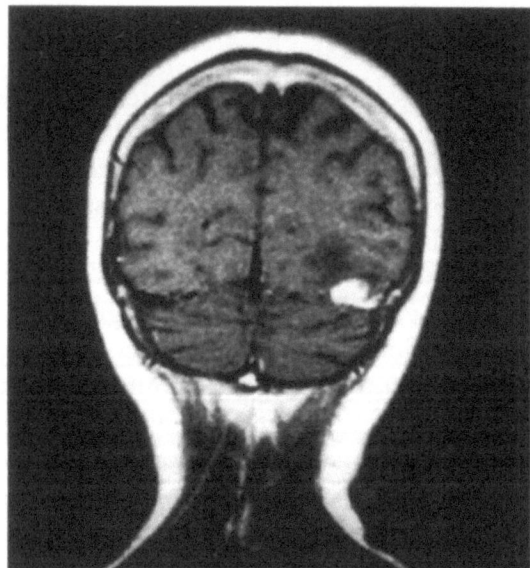

b

Fig. 18a,b Left tentorial meningioma: 10 mm. **a)** Axial T_1-weighted image following i.v. contrast enhancement. **b)** Coronal T_1-weighted image following i.v. contrast enhancement

Acoustic Nerve Neurinoma

Acoustic neurinomas arise from the intracanalicular portion of the nerve; they can extend to the cerebellopontine cistern and compress the pons.

MRI can better detect this tumor and provide an earlier diagnosis than CT, especially if the neurinoma is intracanalicular. On MRI neurinomas appear as roundish lesions with a hypointense signal on T1-weighted images and a hyperintense signal on T2-weighted images. The signal is more intense than that of meningioma and less than that of the cerebral spinal fluid (CSF). After intravenous contrast medium administration, a marked enhancement is present. This can be inhomogeneous because of cystic components that do not exhibit contrast enhancement. Acoustic neurinomas can sometimes be confused with meningiomas, another extra-axial tumor that can localize at the cerebellopontine angle. However, there are some differences: neurinomas extend into the internal auditory canal and have cystic components whereas meningiomas have a dural tail and calcifications.

Trigeminal Neurinoma

Trigeminal neurinomas are diagnosed easily and quite early due to their localization along the nerve pathway, at the prepontine cistern, Meckel's cavity, or upper pars of the cavernous sinus. The signal and enhancement characteristics are similar to those of acoustic neurinomas.

Chordoma

Chordomas are osseous tumors that arise from remnants of the notochord. They are frequently observed in the clivus although the site most frequently involved is the sacrum. Intracranial chordomas appear as an inhomogeneous mass of osseous origin on MRI, extending posteriorly and infiltrating the dura and compressing the brainstem and cerebellum. The signal inhomogeneity is due to cellular and vascular variability of the tumor that presents vascularized areas, calcifications and hemorrhage. Intravenous MRI contrast medium administration produces an irregular and inhomogeneous contrast enhancement. Because of the osseous nature of this tumor the neuroradiological study must be completed with CT of the skull base with a bone window in the axial, coronal, and sagittal planes. Differential diagnosis comprises metastases and chondrosarcoma.

Epidermoid Tumors

Epidermoid tumors are congenital lesions of ectodermal origin. They are covered by a fibrous capsule and lined with a layer of squamous epithelium. They grow slowly and have a very flaky consistency that tends to spread along cleavage planes surrounding the vital structures. The most frequent locations are the cisterns, but they sometimes occur within the ventricles, more commonly the fourth one.

On CT, they present a density similar to that of cerebrospinal fluid (CSF). Differential diagnosis from arachnoid cysts depends on morphological criteria (epidermoid is multilobulate) and location (epidermoid tumors are found in basal cisterns whereas arachnoid cysts are seen in the hemispheric subarachnoid spaces).

On MRI, epidermoid tumors appear as a lesion with intensity similar to that of the CSF, mainly on PD- and T2-weighted images. Diagnosis is made with FLAIR sequences, T2-weighted images, and with selective suppression of the CSF signal. The epidermoid tumors, with these sequences, appear as hyperintense tissue, whereas the CSF presents a hypointense signal. Intravenous contrast medium administration does not enhance these tumors.

Dermoid Tumors

Like epidermoid tumors, dermoid tumors are congenital. They are most frequently localized in the posterior cranial fossa, in the midline, or extend into the supra- and parasellar cisterns; they may also be found in any subarachnoid space or within the ventricles. The appearance of dermoid tumors is characteristic: on MRI they appear as a hyperintense mass on T1-weighted images because of their highly lipidic content, whereas on T2-weighted images they are hypointense. On CT the tumor is characterized by a very low density that is similar to that of adipose tissue. They do not enhance after contrast medium administration.

Germinomas

Germinomas localize in the pineal gland and occur predominantly in males (90% of cases). The peak incidence is during puberty. They tend to spread into the subarachnoid spaces, metastasizing via the CSF. Localization in the suprasellar cisterns is characteristic. On CT and MRI they appear as a mass with a regular border and a roundish lobulated morphology, localized at the level of the pineal gland and which cannot be distinguished from the gland. On MRI the signal intensity is low, similar to that of the gray matter, because of the hypercellularity of the tumor. Peritumoral edema may develop if the tumor infiltrates the surrounding cerebral tissue. After contrast medium administration, a marked and homogeneous enhancement is present, allowing the detection of metastases via CSF.

Pinealomas

Pinealomas affect adults without a sex predilection. On MRI and CT they appear as roundish lesions with well-delimited edges and without infiltration of the adjacent cerebral parenchyma. Pinealomas are characterized by slow growth and, consequently, manifest late. On MRI these tumors appear hypointense on T1-weighted and hyperintense on T2-weighted images. The presence of calcifications and homogeneous enhancement are common features.

Pinealoblastomas

Pinealoblastomas develop from immature, nondifferentiated cells with a high nucleus/cytoplasm ratio and hypercellularity.

Pineoblastomas metastasize in the subarachnoid spaces at an early stage. On MRI this tumor appears as a mass with irregular morphology at the level of the pineal gland with a tendency to infiltrate the surrounding cerebral tissue. Pineoblastomas are characterized by an irregular signal intensity that tends to decrease on T2-weighted images as a result of the hypercellularity. After contrast medium administration a marked and homogeneous enhancement is present.

Colloid Cyst of the Third Ventricle

Colloid cysts are benign tumors arising from neuroepithelial remnants and localized in the anterior part of the third ventricle. These tumors become symptomatic when they occlude the foramen of Monro, causing biventricular hydrocephalus. The content of colloid cysts is different from that of other cystic lesions of the central nervous system, containing mucoid substances, hemoglobin degradation products with macrophages, cholesterol crystals, CSF, and various ions (sodium, magnesium, copper, calcium, phosphorus, and aluminum). The radiological diagnosis is based on the localization, morphology and signal intensity. On MRI colloid cysts appear inhomogeneous. The variability in the signal intensity (marked hypointensity to marked hyperintensity on both T1- and T2-weighted images) depends on the varying content of the cyst and varying concentration of the paramagnetic substances. A thin wall is often present that represents the epithelial layer and that can enhance after contrast administration.

Pituitary Adenomas

MRI is the diagnostic method of choice for studying the sellar region because it allows a study of the gland in the coronal and sagittal planes, which are the most useful for detecting extrasellar extension and involvement of the adjacent structures. Macroadenomas appear hypointense on T1- and hyperintense on T2-weighted images; they displace the pituitary gland, which can be indistinguishable in cases of large adenomas that compress the gland on the floor of the sellar cavity. In macroadenomas cystic components can be present that are seen as roundish, well-circumscribed areas with a hypointense signal on T1- and hyperintense signal on T2-weighted images. After contrast medium administration a marked enhancement is present that can be inhomogeneous if cysts and hemorrhage are present. MRI allows optimal detection of the suprasellar extension of the adenoma, compression on the optic chiasm and third ventricle, and extension toward the sphenoid sinus or cavernous sinuses. If the cavernous sinus is involved, angio-MRI is useful for evaluating the patency of internal carotid arteries, obviating angiography.

MRI is the imaging test of choice to detect microadenoma. It shows a small roundish area located near the pituitary gland. Microadenomas are hypointense on T1- and hyperintense on T2-weighted images compared with the normal glandular parenchyma. Contrast medium administration shows an enhancement of the microadenoma lower than that of normal glandular parenchyma. This finding is sometimes only seen in a dynamic study in an early phase.

Craniopharyngiomas

Craniopharyngiomas represent 3% of cerebral tumors and are located in the sellar region and suprasellar cistern. They have a cystic component and a solid peripheral one. The latter frequently shows calcifications. The content of fluid in the cyst varies, but usually contains cholesterol crystals of variable density and viscosity.

Craniopharyngiomas usually have a characteristic appearance on MRI as an intra-, supra- or retrosellar mass, with an inhomogeneous signal intensity and a roundish central component with well-defined margins. This central component is hyperintense on both T1- and T2-weighted images. In contrast, the peripheral component, often calcified, shows an inhomogeneous signal. After intravenous contrast medium administration a variable enhancement is present at the level of the solid peripheral component.

Lymphomas

Primary central nervous system lymphomas are rare tumors, but are increasing as a result of their frequent association with immunodeficiency syndromes. They occur as intracerebral masses, often multiple and involving the supratentorial structures in 75%-85% of cases. On MRI lymphomas appear as a mass involving the deep gray matter, periventricular regions, and corpus callosum. Generally there is no perilesional edema, calcification, or hemorrhage.

Usually, the signal is isointense compared to gray matter on all the sequences, particularly when the lymphoma involves deep gray matter structures, but sometimes they can be hyperintense on PD- and T2-weighted images. Contrast enhancement is usually marked and homogeneous. Contrast-enhanced MRI is very useful in detecting meningeal involvement in cases of metastases from systemic lymphoma. Differential diagnosis encompasses metastases and inflammatory disease, i.e., toxoplasmosis, in AIDS cases. It is reported that in patients affected by AIDS lymphoma can present as multiple lesions with perilesional edema and peripheral enhancement.

Metastases

Intra-axial

Contrast-enhanced MRI is better than CT in the detection of these lesions. Metastases appear as solid nodules of varying signal intensity, but often hyperintense on PD- and T2-weighted images. The edema feature can be helpful in distinguishing solitary metastases from primitive tumors of the central nervous system.

The variability in signal of the metastatic nodule depends on the pathological changes in the tumor. Necrotic components appear hyperintense on T2- and hypointense on T1-weighted images. Hemorrhages show the characteristic signal of hemoglobin degradation products. Metastases from melanoma without hemorrhage present a particular signal: hyperintense on T1- and isointense on T2-

weighted images. Most cerebral metastases demonstrate contrast enhancement, which can appear as solid or nodular or with an irregular ring.

Differential diagnosis encompasses glioblastoma and abscess.

Extra-axial

Epidural metastases are usually due to the presence of metastasis of the cranial theca. Subdural metastases are due to hematogenous spread. Primitive tumors, adenocarcinomas, melanomas, leukemia, and lymphoma can spread into the subarachnoid spaces. MRI shows marked enhancement of the leptomeninges and sometimes of the ependymal surfaces.